Prevention Strategies after
Myocardial Infarction

second edition

JGF Cleland

British Heart Foundation Fellow
MRC Clinical Research
Initiative in Heart Failure
University of Glasgow, UK

SG Ray

Senior Registrar in Cardiology
Cardiothoracic Centre
Liverpool, UK

JJV McMurray

Department of Cardiology
Western General Hospital
Edinburgh, UK

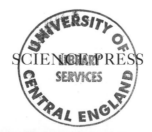

SCIENCE PRESS

Published by Science Press Limited, 34–42 Cleveland Street, London W1P 6LB, UK

www.science-press.com

© Science Press Ltd 1994, 1997

First published 1994

Second edition 1997

British Library Cataloguing-in-Publication data.

A catalogue record for this book is available from the British Library.

ISBN 1-85873-252-2

Although every effort has been made to ensure that drug doses and other inform-ation are presented accurately in this publication, the ultimate responsibility rests with the prescribing physician. Neither the publisher nor the authors can be held responsible for errors or for any consequences arising from the use of information contained herein. Any product mentioned in this publication should be used in accordance with the prescribing information prepared by the manufacturers. No claims or endorsements are made for any drug or compound at present under clini-cal investigation.

Project editor: Amanda Tyndall
Indexer: Dr Olivera Potparic
Illustrator: Mathew McCutcheon
Typesetter: Paul Angliss
Designer: Claire Huntley
Production controller: Yolanda Perez Capilla

Printed in Singapore by Stamford Press

Contents

Trial acronyms

4S Scandinavian Simvastatin Survival Study

AIMS APSAC Intervention Mortality Study

AIRE Acute Infarction Ramipril Efficacy

AMIS Aspirin Myocardial Infarction Study

APSI Acebutolol et Prévention Secondaire de l'Infarctus (Acebutolol and secondary prevention of infarction)

ASPECT Anticoagulants in the Secondary Prevention of Events in Coronary Thrombosis

ASSET Anglo-Scandinavian Study of Early Thrombolysis

BASIS Basel Antiarrhythmic Study of Infarct Survival

BHAT Beta blocker Heart Attack research group

CAST Cardiac Arrhythmia Suppression Trial

CDP Coronary Drug Project

CONSENSUS Cooperative North Scandinavian Enalapril Survival Study

CSBG European Coronary Bypass Group

DART Diet and Reinfarction Trial

DIGAMI Diabetic patients receiving Insulin-Glucose infusion during Acute Myocardial Infarction

DAVIT Danish Verapamil Infarction Trial

EAMI Exercise in Anterior Myocardial Infarction

ECSG European Cooperative Study Group for t-PA in acute myocardial infarction

EIS European Infarction Study

EMERAS Estudio Multicentrico Estreptoquinasa Republicas de Americas del Sur (multicentre streptokinase study)

EMIP European Myocardial Infarction Project

EPSIM Enquête de Prévention Secondaire de l'Infarctus du Myocarde (secondary prevention of myocardial infarction research group)

ESPRIM European Study Prevention Research of Infarct with Moisidomine

ESVEM Electrophysiologic Study Versus Electrocardiographic Monitoring

GAMIS German-Austrian Myocardial Infarction Study

GISSI Gruppo Italiano per lo Studio Sopravvivenza nell'Infarto miocardio (Italian study group on streptokinase in myocardial infarction)

GREAT Grampian Region Early Anistreplase Trial

GUSTO Global Utilization of Streptokinase and Tissue plasminogen activator for Occluded coronary arteries

IMPACT International Mexiletine and Placebo Antiarrhythmic Coronary Trial

ISIS International Study of Infarct Survival

LATE Late Assessment of Thrombolytic Efficacy

LIMIT Leicester Intravenous Magnesium Intervention Trial

LIT Lopressor Intervention Trial

MDPIT Mulicentre Diltiazem Post Infarction Trial research group

Trial acronyms *(continued)*

MIAMI Metoprolol In Acute Myocardial Infarction

MITI Myocardial Infarction Triage and Intervention trial

MPIP Multicentre Post Infarction Program

N-NLIT North-Norwegian Lidocaine Intervention Trial

PARIS Persantin-Aspirin Reinfarction Study

PRACTICAL Placebo-controlled Random Angiotensin-converting enzyme inhibition Comparative Trial In Cardiac infarction and Left ventricular function

PREMIS PREmenopausal Morphometric Intervention Study

QUIET QUinapril Ischaemic Event Trial

RISK Risk Intervention SKills study

SAVE Survival And Ventricular Enlargement study

SCATI Studio sulla Calciparina nell'Angina e nella Trombosi ventricolare nell'Infarto (study of calciparine in angina, ventricular thrombosis and infarction)

SMILE Survival of Myocardial Infarction Long-term Evaluation

SOLVD Studies Of Left Ventricular Dysfunction

SPRINT Secondary Prevention Reinfarction Israeli Nifedipine Trial

SWIFT Should We Intervene Following Thrombolysis?

TAMI Transmural Anterior Myocardial Infarction

TIMI Thrombolysis in Myocardial Infarction

TOPS Treatment Of Post-thrombolytic Stenosis

TRACE TRAndolopril Cardiac Evaluation

TRENT TRial of Early Nifedipine Treatment in acute myocardial infarction

WARIS WArfarin ReInfarction Study

WASH Warfarin/Aspirin Study of Heart failure

Abbreviations

ACE angiotensin-converting enzyme

AMI acute myocardial infarction

ANP atrial natriuretic peptide

APSAC anisoylated plasminogen streptokinase activator complex

AVP arginine vasopressin

BNP brain natriuretic peptide

BRS baroreflex sensitivity

CABG coronary artery bypass graft

CCU coronary care unit

CHF chronic heart failure

CVA cerebrovascular accident

ECG electrocardiogram

ESV end-systolic volume

ETT exercise tolerance test

GIK glucose-insulin-potassium

GP general practitioner

HRV heart rate variability

INR International Normalized Ratio

ISA intrinsic sympathomimetic activity

IV intravenous

LV left ventricular

LVEDP left ventricular end-diastolic pressure

LVEDV left ventricular end-diastolic volume

LVEF left ventricular ejection fraction

LVF left ventricular failure

METs metabolic equivalents

MI myocardial infarction

MR mitral regurgitation

MRC Medical Research Council

MU mega units

ns non-significant

PC (radiological) pulmonary congestion

PES programmed electrical stimulation

PNS parasympathetic nervous system

PTCA percutaneous transluminal coronary angioplasty

R.Excess R relative excess risk

RNVG radionuclide ventriculography

RRR relative risk reduction

SAECG signal averaged ECG

SC subcutaneous

SK streptokinase

SNS sympathetic nervous system

tPA (recombinant) tissue plasminogen activator

u units

VEB ventricular ectopic beat

VF ventricular fibrillation

VT ventricular tachycardia

WHO World Health Organization

CHAPTER 1

Cardiovascular adaptation and maladaptation after myocardial infarction

Simon Ray and John GF Cleland

Acute myocardial infarction (AMI) produces a dramatic change in the mechanical and biochemical influences exerted on the heart, leading to complex and imperfectly understood changes both in infarcted and in surviving myocardium.

Infarct zone remodelling

Myocardial infarction (MI) results in impaired systolic contraction and a rise in end-diastolic volume and pressure, which leads to passive stretch of the myocardium. The consequent increase in myocardial wall stress (*see* Figure 1.1) causes myocytes in the infarcted area to slide over one another, thus thinning the infarct zone and increasing its surface area — known as infarct expansion [1,2]. The distortion of ventricular shape and the increase in chamber radius due to infarct expansion increase wall stress in the non-infarcted myocardium, which undergoes eccentric hypertrophy. The myocardial collagen fibres that would normally prevent this expansion are damaged by collagenase, which is released in response to ischaemia and inflammation [3]. Infarct expansion may be detected on the echocardiogram as early as two hours after

Figure 1.1.
(a) The average circumferential wall stress (force per unit of cross-sectional area of wall) is related directly to the product of intra-ventricular pressure and chamber radius (r) and related inversely to wall thickness (w).
(b) In compensated hypertrophy, there is ventricular enlargement but the ratio of chamber radius to wall thickness is preserved (i.e., $r^1/w^1 \approx r/w$) and wall stress is therefore relatively normal at rest.
(c) If the dilatation is proportionately greater than wall thickening (i.e., $r^2/w^2 > r/w$) then wall stress will remain chronically elevated and dilatation may be progressive.

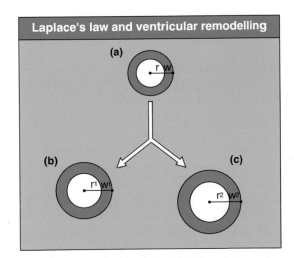

Laplace's law and ventricular remodelling

the onset of symptoms [4]. It is restricted to transmural infarcts, is greater in anterior infarcts and is proportional to infarct size [5]. In extreme cases, expansion may lead to cardiac rupture. Shortly after infarction, macrophages migrate to the infarct zone to lyse necrotic myocytes; fibroblasts also migrate there and produce new collagen fibres. The collagen content of the infarct increases to five times normal levels over a six-week period, resulting in a stable, stretch-resistant scar with some contraction of the infarct zone [6].

Infarcts are not homogeneous masses of necrotic tissue but may contain islands of viable cells towards the periphery. This may be an important factor in limiting the extent of infarct expansion. In addition, the routine use of thrombolytic agents has changed the pathology of MI by increasing the proportion of viable myocardium within the infarcted area.

Global ventricular remodelling

The architecture of the remaining functioning myocardium is remodelled from the molecular level upwards. The central stimulus to remodelling is the abnormally high mechanical stress imposed on the remaining viable myocytes by the sudden stretching of the myocardium as diastolic pressure and volume rise, and the infarct zone is distorted and expanded [7,8]. Wall stress increases with the degree of infarct expansion and is particularly high in the areas bordering the infarct zone. Myocyte slippage occurs in the viable myocardium as a result of the high wall stress, but cellular hypertrophy is the major cause of chronic global ventricular dilatation [9]. Stretch-sensitive ion channels in the cell membrane stimulate protein synthesis and formation of new sarcomeres, augmented by the trophic effects of growth factors such as angiotensin II and by the sympathetic nervous system (SNS) [8,10]. The result is eccentric hypertrophy, predominantly through an increase in the length but also in the width of individual myocytes, reflected in chamber enlargement and an increase in wall thickness (*see* Figure 1.2) [9]. In the short term, chamber enlargement can be advantageous. Stretching of the viable myocardium increases the force of contraction via the Frank–Starling mechanism, and with a larger chamber the same stroke volume can be ejected with proportionately less contraction of individual myocytes (*see* Figure 1.2). However, this short-term gain is achieved at the cost of a further increase in wall stress, particularly in diastole, which may be harmful in the long term [7,9].

After experimental infarcts involving less than 40% of left ventricular (LV) mass, a state of compensated eccentric hypertrophy can develop where the hypertrophy of the remaining viable myocytes is sufficient to restore ventricular mass to near-normal levels [9]. The increase in width of the hypertrophied myocytes, and hence the increase in wall thickness, is sufficient to offset the increase in diastolic wall stress caused by their lengthening and the corresponding increase in chamber radius (*see* Figure 1.1). In large infarcts (involving about 60% of ventricular mass) cellular

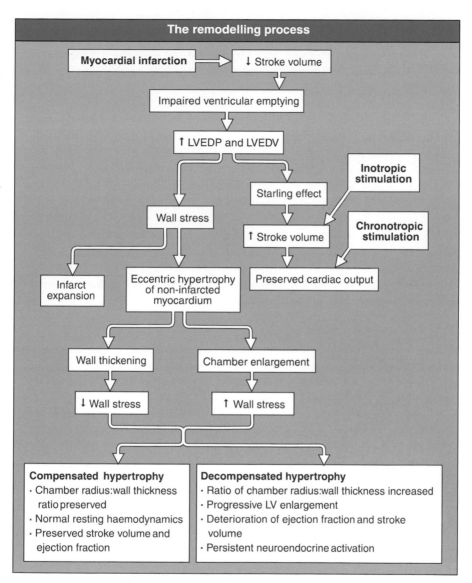

Figure 1.2. Schematic outline of the remodelling process. Impaired ventricular emptying (decreased stroke volume) increases end-diastolic volume and pressure, stretching the non-infarcted myocardium. Diastolic stretch increases the force of contraction — known as the Starling effect — and returns stroke volume towards normal. This effect is augmented by the positive inotropic and chronotropic effects of sympathoadrenergic stimulation. The increase in diastolic volume that initiates the Starling effect is accompanied by an increase in wall stress (see Figure 1.1), which initiates infarct expansion and eccentric hypertrophy. In patients with large infarcts, eccentric hypertrophy may become decompensated and result in progressive ventricular dysfunction. LVEDP, left ventricular end-diastolic pressure; LVEDV, left ventricular end-diastolic volume; LV, left ventricular.

hypertrophy is insufficient to restore ventricular mass, despite a quantitatively greater increase in the size of individual myocytes [9]. The increase in cell width is insufficient to counteract the effects of cell lengthening and slippage, and the ratio of chamber radius to wall thickness is increased by about 20%. In this situation, the mechanical stress of the remaining myocytes is persistently high and may lead to progressive ventricular dilatation [7,9] (*see* Figures 1.1 and 1.2).

Hypertrophied myocytes from dilating ventricles do not function normally since contraction and relaxation are abnormally slow [11]. The formation of abnormal contractile proteins, abnormalities of mitochondrial enzymes or a decrease in the ratio of mitochondria to myofibrils may play a role in this slowing [8].

The collagenous structure of the viable myocardium is also remodelled in the failing ventricle [12]. Distortion of the intricate collagen network and excessive fibrosis may make the remodelled ventricle less compliant, impairing diastolic filling [13]. Capillary density is reduced within remodelled myocardium [9], and coronary flow reserve is impaired [14]. Relative underperfusion may contribute further to myocardial depression and excessive fibrosis, and may provide the substrate for ventricular dysrhythmias. Chronic structural modifications that may occur in remodelling myocardium are outlined in Figure 1.3.

Factors influencing remodelling

Factors known to influence the extent of ventricular remodelling are listed in Table 1.1. Patency of the infarct-related artery plays an important role. Acute reperfusion reverses the early infarct expansion that is already present on admission, and thus limits subsequent global remodelling [15]. Spontaneous reperfusion that is too late to salvage infarcting myocardium also limits dilatation [16], whereas clinically silent late reocclusion of an initially patent artery is associated with a deterioration in cardiac function [17]. Patients with persisting occlusion and no collateral flow show the most marked dilatation [18]. In this situation, it is uncertain whether persistent occlusion of the infarct-related artery *per se* is the major cause of remodelling, or whether persistent occlusion is simply a result of the lack of a sufficient metabolic stimulus to maintain arterial patency to a large and total transmural infarct zone.

The benefit of acute reperfusion is probably the result of decreased infarct transmurality, that is, the preservation of a rim or islands of functioning myocytes and collagen on the epicardial surface [15], which may act as a restraint against cell slippage and reduce transmural stress. The effect of late reperfusion is less certain but it does not appear to alter the collagen content or the tensile strength of the scar [19]. The presence of anterograde flow in the infarct zone might increase tissue turgor, stiffen the myocardium and thus limit dilatation. Improvement of cardiac function after late reperfusion can occur rapidly, suggesting that viable but non-functioning (hibernating) myocardium might be recruited by the improved blood supply [15,20].

Diabetic patients are more likely to develop heart failure after AMI than are

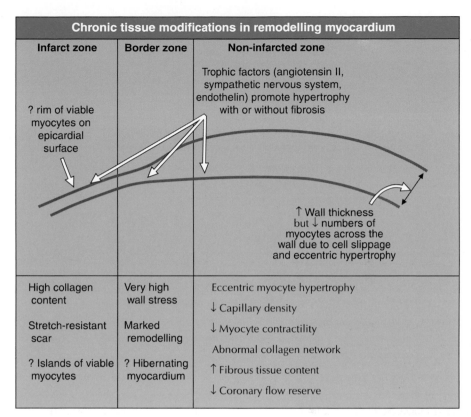

Chronic tissue modifications in remodelling myocardium		
Infarct zone	**Border zone**	**Non-infarcted zone**
High collagen content	Very high wall stress	Eccentric myocyte hypertrophy
		↓ Capillary density
Stretch-resistant scar	Marked remodelling	↓ Myocyte contractility
		Abnormal collagen network
? Islands of viable myocytes	? Hibernating myocardium	↑ Fibrous tissue content
		↓ Coronary flow reserve

Within figure: ? rim of viable myocytes on epicardial surface

Trophic factors (angiotensin II, sympathetic nervous system, endothelin) promote hypertrophy with or without fibrosis

↑ Wall thickness but ↓ numbers of myocytes across the wall due to cell slippage and eccentric hypertrophy

Figure 1.3. There is a gradual transition from infarcted to non-infarcted zones through a border zone that probably contains hibernating myocardium and that is subject to particularly high levels of stress. Trophic factors affect the remodelling of all three zones. All myocardial changes are more pronounced in patients with decompensated hypertrophy.

non-diabetic patients with infarcts of similar size [21]. The mechanisms involved are uncertain but may be related to myocardial small vessel disease.

Clinical correlates of remodelling

Patients with transmural infarcts and LV dysfunction, but no overt heart failure, may be divided into three groups [22].

- About 55% show no significant ventricular enlargement since insufficient myocardium is lost to trigger any measurable remodelling.
- In 25%, limited ventricular enlargement is seen in the first six months, followed by stabilization of end-systolic volume and a small decrease in end-diastolic volume. Here, left ventricular ejection fraction (LVEF) is stable in the long term. These patients are the clinical correlate of compensated eccentric hypertrophy, where remodelling helps to restore stroke volume and preserve exercise capacity.

Factors influencing the extent of ventricular remodelling
Inhibition Patency of the infarct-related artery, irrespective of the time of reperfusion Collateral flow to the infarct zone
Exacerbation Increased infarct size Anterior infarct Extensive early infarct expansion Persistent occlusion or reocclusion of the infarct-related artery without collaterals Steroids Non-steroidal anti-inflammatory drugs Diabetes

Table 1.1.

- In 20% of patients, ventricular size increases progressively from admission. Initially, dilatation is compensatory and the larger chamber allows for preservation of stroke volume but, with continuing enlargement, stroke volume and ejection fraction begin to decline after approximately six months [22]. As ventricular remodelling progresses, the cavity becomes more spherical, distorting further normal coordinated contraction, increasing wall stress and worsening cardiac mechanics [23]. Distortion of ventricular shape also predisposes to mitral regurgitation. Increased end-systolic volume is a very powerful predictor of late prognosis after MI [24].

Circulatory adaptation

Circulatory adaptation to MI is inextricably linked to cardiac function and activation of the neuroendocrine axis. In the acute phase, patients with large LV infarcts have low systemic arterial pressures, raised filling pressures and raised systemic vascular resistance [25]. These changes persist in patients with continuing heart failure. Chronically, patients in the group with no detectable ventricular remodelling have normal central haemodynamics at rest and a normal response to exercise [22]. Resting haemodynamics are normal in those with limited remodelling but there is a progressive rise in pulmonary wedge pressure on exercise, that is, the Frank–Starling mechanism is necessary to maintain stroke volume during exercise. In patients with progressive ventricular enlargement, wedge pressure rises, initially on exercise but subsequently at rest, and systemic vascular resistance increases as heart failure develops. Overt heart failure is characterized by markedly impaired ventriculo-arterial coupling [26], reduced renal and superior mesenteric blood flow, and impaired flow to skeletal muscle during exercise [27].

The progression of these abnormalities in patients with asymptomatic LV dysfunction has not been well characterized, but renal vasoconstriction is present for at least six months in patients with moderate to large anterior infarcts [28].

Neuroendocrine activation

Significant transmural MI causes a sudden reduction in ventricular stroke volume and cardiac output, which are sensed by arterial baroreceptors, triggering a nonspecific vasoconstrictor, antidiuretic and antinatriuretic response (*see* Table 1.2) [29]. Superimposed on this response are the effects of pain, nausea, drug treatment and elevation of LV end-diastolic, atrial and pulmonary pressures (*see* Figure 1.4).

The sympathoadrenergic system

Plasma concentrations of adrenaline and noradrenaline are elevated in most patients admitted to coronary care units (CCUs) with chest pain [30]. In those with uncomplicated infarcts, admission levels of both hormones approximate to those seen in healthy subjects during moderate exercise and usually decline to the normal range

The effects of neuroendocrine activation in acute MI	
Renin–angiotensin system Coronary vasoconstriction Peripheral vasoconstriction Decreased venous capacitance Increased myocardial contractility Sodium and water retention Renal potassium loss Potentiation of sympathetic neurotransmission Direct cardiac toxicity Stimulation of fibroblast activity	**Arginine vasopressin** Coronary vasoconstriction Peripheral vasoconstriction Water retention **Endothelin** Coronary vasoconstriction Peripheral vasoconstriction Decreased venous capacitance Increased myocardial contractility Sodium retention

Sympathoadrenal system
Increased myocardial contractility
Tachycardia
Coronary vasoconstriction
Peripheral vasoconstriction
Decreased venous capacitance
Arrhythmogenesis
Metabolic effects:
    Increased free fatty acids
    Hypokalaemia
    Potentiation of eccentric hypertrophy
    Direct cardiac toxicity
	Atrial natriuretic peptide
	Coronary vasodilatation
	Peripheral vasodilatation
	Increased venous capacitance
	Inhibition of vasoconstrictor mechanisms
	Possible negative inotropic properties
	Diuresis
	Natriuresis
	
	Brain natriuretic peptide
	Peripheral vasodilatation
	Diuresis
	Natriuresis
	Inhibition of vasoconstrictor mechanisms

Table 1.2.

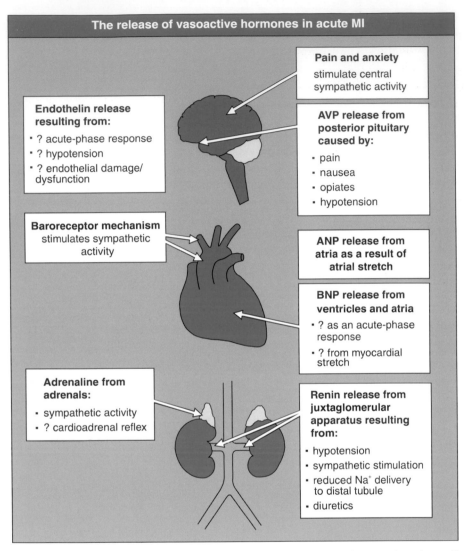

Figure 1.4. Numerous interrelated factors stimulate the release of vasoactive hormones in patients with myocardial infarction. Individual hormones do not act in isolation and fluctuations in the levels of one hormone influence the release and activity of others. Release of other hormones may also be influenced by myocardial infarction (e.g. thyroid hormones and insulin). AVP, arginine vasopressin; ANP, atrial natriuretic peptide; BNP, brain natriuretic peptide.

within 24–48 hours [30]. In patients with cardiogenic shock, concentrations reach levels similar to those seen with phaeochromocytoma and may remain elevated [30,31]. Although pain and associated anxiety are important factors in catecholamine release, plasma levels are higher in uncomplicated infarcts than in patients with ischaemic chest pain and no infarct; thus, other mechanisms must also be involved [30].

A reduction in cardiac output or a change in the aortic pressure waveform probably stimulates a reflex increase in sympathetic activity, mediated by arterial baroreceptors [29]. Cardiac sympathetic activity is also increased by local cardio-cardiac reflexes in response to tissue acidosis and myocardial wall stress [32]. Adrenal secretion of adrenaline may also be increased by stimulation of cardiac receptors [33].

Autonomic tone is disturbed following MI. Studies of heart rate variability (HRV) indicate that cardiac sympathetic activity is increased and cardiac parasympathetic activity is decreased for about one year [34]. Baroreflex sensitivity (BRS) is also reduced soon after infarction, increasing to normal values at about three months post-infarct [35]. Both reduced HRV and reduced BRS reflect decreased cardiac parasympathetic activity and are predictive of dysrhythmic events and death.

The renin–angiotensin system

The renin–angiotensin system (*see* Figure 1.5) is strikingly activated in patients given diuretics for cardiac failure, but is also activated in patients with LV dysfunction who do not receive diuretics [30]. Plasma renin activity in this group is about twice that in normal controls 12 days after infarction [36]. Peak levels both of renin and of angiotensin II occur at about 72 hours after admission, irrespective of diuretic treatment [30]. In patients treated with diuretics, angiotensin levels reach eight times the upper limit of normal; nevertheless, several factors other than diuretic use contribute to the activation of the renin–angiotensin system after AMI. Increased sympathetic

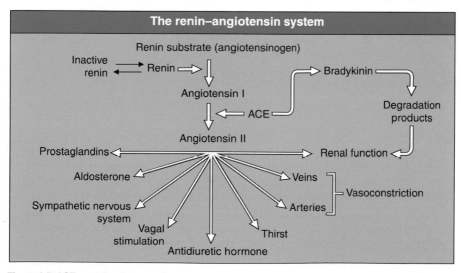

Figure 1.5. ACE, angiotensin-converting enzyme.

nervous activity and raised levels of circulating catecholamines stimulate renin secretion from the renal juxtaglomerular apparatus, as does the reduction in renal perfusion pressure that occurs with systemic hypotension [37]. All of these are more likely to occur in patients with larger infarcts and greater degrees of LV dysfunction. In a multivariate analysis of 519 patients 12 days post-infarction, plasma renin activity was significantly related only to diuretic use and LVEF [36]. The relevance of activation of the renin–angiotensin system to ventricular remodelling is further supported by the beneficial effects of angiotensin-converting enzyme (ACE) inhibitors observed post-infarction.

Endothelin

Plasma concentrations of endothelin are elevated after AMI, with peak levels of two to five times normal within six hours of admission, even in patients with no clinically detectable haemodynamic disturbance [38]. In uncomplicated infarcts, plasma levels decline to normal within 72 hours of admission, but in patients with cardiogenic shock, peak levels rise as high as 14 times normal, remaining elevated for at least several days [39]. The stimuli to endothelin release in AMI are uncertain. Several factors have been proposed, including activation of the coagulation system [40], damage to the coronary endothelium, myocardial hypoxia and hypotension [41]. Another possibility is that endothelin is part of a non-specific acute-phase response and the human pre-proendothelin-1 gene contains sequences related to the acute-phase reactant response [42]. The very high levels in patients with cardiogenic shock may be the result of multi-organ ischaemia, generalized endothelial dysfunction or reduced renal clearance of endothelin [43].

Arginine vasopressin

Plasma arginine vasopressin (AVP) is markedly elevated early after infarction despite a decrease in osmolality. Levels in most patients decline to normal over about three days. In the SAVE study, 27% of patients had persistently high plasma levels at 12 days post-infarct [36].

Atrial natriuretic peptide

Plasma concentrations of atrial natriuretic peptide (ANP) are increased between two- and three-fold as early as 45 minutes after the onset of AMI [44]. This is followed, within four hours of admission, by a fall to concentrations within the normal range, and then by a secondary rise at 24–48 hours when concentrations reach 75–100% of those on admission [45,46]. This pattern is observed both in complicated and in uncomplicated infarcts but the secondary rise is much more prominent in patients in Killip class 2 or above [46]. In patients without heart failure, plasma concentrations of ANP remain at or just above the upper limit of normal for at least one month after infarction [47]. In those with heart failure, levels are persistently raised at around two to three times the upper limit of normal [47]. The sudden rise in plasma ANP after MI is caused by atrial distension as a result of ventricular dysfunction. The subsequent fall and secondary rise in levels may result from exhaustion of atrial storage granules by the initial surge of release, followed by synthesis of new hormone, which restores circulating concentrations to supranormal levels [45]. ANP is synthesized in ventricular myocardium in patients who develop cardiac failure [48].

Brain natriuretic peptide

Brain natriuretic peptide (BNP) is a cardiac hormone secreted predominantly from ventricular myocardium [46]. Plasma levels increase 60-fold after AMI, peaking at around 20 hours. In patients with small uncomplicated infarcts, the concentration declines steadily over several days but remains many times normal values for at least one month in patients with large or complicated infarcts [46]. At plasma levels similar to those in patients with mild cardiac failure, BNP has natriuretic and vasodilator effects [49]. The initial peak in BNP may be an acute-phase response but the persistently high levels in patients with large infarcts probably reflect the ventricular wall stress related to ventricular dilatation [46]. For this reason, a sustained rise in BNP may prove to be a good marker for ventricular remodelling.

Bradykinin and prostacyclins

There is some evidence for the production of vasodilator kinins and prostacyclins in AMI [50,51]. They and nitric oxide probably play a role in the modulation of vascular tone but their importance is uncertain. ACE inhibitors may prevent the degradation of bradykinin, which may, in turn, stimulate production of nitric oxide and vasodilator prostaglandins. The importance of this pathway for the effects of ACE inhibition is unclear.

Influence of the neuroendocrine response to myocardial infarction

---

The net action of the neuroendocrine response to MI is vasoconstrictor, antinatriuretic and antidiuretic. The extent of activation varies widely between patients and cannot wholly be explained by LV dysfunction or diuretic use [36]. In the SAVE study 48% of patients with asymptomatic LV dysfunction had activation of at least one vasoconstrictor hormone 12 days post-infarct [36]. In some patients, this hormonal activation becomes chronic and may contribute to the progression of ventricular enlargement [52]. ANP and BNP counteract the effects of vasoconstrictor hormones and may be endogenous modulators of progressive ventricular dilatation. By reducing cardiac filling pressures, they reduce diastolic wall stress, which is the major stimulus to ventricular dilatation. In patients from the SAVE study, 61% had elevated levels of ANP at 12 days post–infarct [36]. Plasma ANP measured at three days is an independent predictor of late survival, probably a reflection of its relationship to ventricular filling pressures and thus ventricular dysfunction [53].

Effects of ACE inhibitors on remodelling and sudden death

Recent studies suggest that ACE inhibitors delay or prevent the onset of heart failure requiring diuretic therapy in selected patients immediately after AMI or in those with chronic LV dysfunction [54,55]. To what extent does remodelling account for the beneficial effects of ACE inhibitors?

Effects of interventions other than ACE inhibitors on LV remodelling

After AMI, a favourable effect of nitrates on remodelling [56] has not been supported by recent large trials [57,58]. Loop diuretics [59] and digoxin [60] do not alter remodelling favourably, while magnesium [58,61] and calcium antagonists [62,63] do not reduce the risk of developing heart failure after AMI. Beta blockers reduce the risk of developing heart failure in selected patients after AMI [64], and can improve haemodynamics and increase ejection fraction in patients with dilated cardiomyopathy [65]. Revascularization may result in marked improvements in volume and function in selected patients [66].

Effects of ACE inhibitors on LV volume and ejection fraction

ACE inhibitors reduce LV volumes after AMI, mostly by limiting the extent of infarct zone expansion [67], especially anterior infarct, with lesser effects on dilatation of the non-infarct zone (*see* Table 1.3).

The SAVE study reported beneficial effects of captopril in reducing LV end-systolic and end-diastolic areas when an ACE inhibitor was initiated an average of 11 days after AMI [68]. However, the benefit was small compared with the obvious clinical benefit. Infarct expansion occurs most rapidly early after AMI and a greater effect in reducing infarct expansion is observed if the ACE inhibitor is started early rather than late [59,69].

The CONSENSUS II study showed that the beneficial effect of ACE inhibitors on cardiac volumes was obvious at four weeks, with little further effect after six months of randomized therapy [70]. Although mortality was not reduced, a significant reduction in heart failure did occur. A placebo cross-over study by Bazzino *et al.* showed that an ACE inhibitor initiated two months, after AMI had little effect on cardiac volumes in the subsequent two months, while an ACE inhibitor started soon after AMI had pronounced effects that persisted even after the drug's withdrawal [71].

The GISSI-III study confirmed the beneficial effects of early treatment with lisinopril in reducing the number of patients with an ejection fraction <35% at six weeks post-infarction, though this did not translate at this early stage into a reduction in clinical heart failure [57]. At six weeks, patients were withdrawn from randomized therapy and patients with a definite indication for an ACE inhibitor could be treated accordingly. Patients were followed until six months, at which time it appeared that the early benefit of lisinopril on LV function had been largely main-

Mechanisms by which ACE inhibitors may reduce progressive ventricular dilatation
• Reduction in ventricular pre- and after-load
• Resetting of ventricular volumes (possibly secondary to the above)
• Remodelling (secondary to haemodynamic and neuro-endocrine effects)
• Reduction in recurrent ischaemia/infarction

Figure 1.3. ACE, angiotensin-converting enzyme.

tained despite withdrawal of the drug (GISSI-III: Oral communication from the European Society of Cardiology Meeting on Heart Failure, Glasgow, 1994).

The SOLVD studies demonstrated that enalapril reduced LV volumes for up to four years [72–74]. However, the largest change in volume occurred in the first four months, with little additional effect thereafter. This effect might be termed "resetting" rather than remodelling [75], the latter implying a process of continuing improvement. However, the change in LV volumes was not solely due to a haemodynamic effect of enalapril, as LV volumes were reduced, compared with placebo, after withdrawing the ACE inhibitor.

Effects of ACE inhibitors on LV hypertrophy, myocardial fibrosis and compliance

ACE inhibitors reduce concentric hypertrophy in hypertension [76], but the effect on the eccentric hypertrophy that occurs after AMI is less clear.

The SOLVD study indicated that enalapril prevented LV mass from increasing further in patients with chronic LV dysfunction [74]. The preferential and earlier reduction in volume means that the mass/volume ratio increases, reducing wall stress.

Animal studies suggest that angiotensin II induces fibroblast proliferation and increases collagen synthesis, and that ACE inhibitors may modify favourably the accumulation of collagen and myocardial fibrosis in experimental LV hypertrophy and post-infarction myocardium [77,78]. The relevance of these findings to human disease is yet to be determined. There is no evidence of an adverse effect of ACE inhibitors on collagen deposition required to produce a stable scar after MI. Indeed, ACE inhibitors appear to exert a major part of their benefits by reducing scar "stretch" [67].

Myocardial compliance is decreased in heart failure but LV compliance is paradoxically increased because of the higher wall stress. The SOLVD study suggests that long-term ACE inhibition reduces filling pressures to a lesser extent than LV diastolic volume [79], implying that ACE inhibitors reduce LV compliance towards normal. ACE inhibitors used acutely after AMI improve Doppler filling

13

characteristics in the long term [80], possibly because of effects on LV remodelling
and changes in loading conditions.

Effects of ACE inhibitors on peripheral vascular structure

In heart failure, maximal vasodilatation induced by drugs or metabolic stress is
reduced, suggesting that structural changes may be important in regulating blood-
flow [81]. Alveolar–capillary membrane dysfunction in heart failure may represent
similar structural changes in the pulmonary vasculature [82]. Although ACE
inhibitors reduce vascular resistance both at rest and during exercise, it is unclear
how much of this is due to a beneficial effect on vascular remodelling.

Effects of ACE inhibitors on salt and water balance

Patients with heart failure commonly retain salt and water in the first few days after
starting an ACE inhibitor [83], though this is usually self-limiting and reverses
spontaneously [84,85]. Only two out of eleven placebo-controlled studies that measured long-term changes in weight noted a decline, suggesting diuresis.

Effects of ACE inhibitors on arrhythmias, recurrent infarction and sudden death

Several studies [84–88] suggest that ACE inhibitors reduce arrhythmias in heart failure
and after AMI, but the SOLVD study was unable to confirm this fact [89]. ACE
inhibitors improve LV loading, reduce volumes and retard progressive hypertrophy,
increase serum potassium and improve autonomic balance, and so they should reduce
arrhythmias [90]. Studies of ACE inhibitors in human heart failure have suggested
only subtle electrophysiological effects, which may, however, be important [91].

Recurrent infarction causes further LV damage and confers a greater risk of
developing heart failure or dying [92,93]. A beneficial effect of ACE inhibitors on
recurrent ischaemic events may be an important effect on chronic LV function. The
QUIET study, which is investigating the effects of quinapril on recurrent ischaemic
events in patients with coronary disease but no substantial LV dysfunction, will be
critical in resolving these arguments.

Many studies have suggested that ACE inhibitors reduce sudden death [94–97],
secondary to a reduction in either arrhythmias or AMI. The CONSENSUS [98] and
the SOLVD [99] treatment trials are the exceptions, both suggesting a predominant
effect of ACE inhibitors on progressive heart failure deaths. Anomalies in reporting
probably account for the differences between studies [100]. Enalapril reduced
mortality during the run-in period in the SOLVD study [99], which, in the context of
a randomized trial in stable patients, implies a reduction in sudden unexpected death.

In summary, there is no doubt that ACE inhibitors reduce LV volumes, but
whether the principal reason for this is an acute resetting of volumes mediated
primarily through reduced haemodynamic stress, retardation of progressive remodelling through alterations in LV stress and inhibition of neuroendocrine activation,
or prevention of recurrent ischaemic damage to the left ventricle is unclear.

References

1. Hutchins GM, Bulkley BH: **Infarct expansion versus extension: two different complications of acute myocardial infarction.** *Am J Cardiol* 1978, **41**:1127–1132.

2. Weissman HF *et al.*: **Cellular mechanisms of myocardial infarct expansion.** *Circulation* 1988, **78**:186–201.

3. Whittaker P *et al.*: **Role of collagen in acute myocardial infarct expansion.** *Circulation* 1991, **84**:2123–2134.

4. Picard M *et al.*: **Natural history of LV size and function after acute myocardial infarction.** *Circulation* 1990, **82**:484–494.

5. Pfeffer MA, Braunwald E: **Ventricular remodelling after myocardial infarction.** *Circulation* 1990, **81**:1161–1172.

6. Sato S *et al.*: **Connective tissue changes in early ischaemia of porcine myocardium: an ultrastructural study.** *J Mol Cell Cardiol* 1983, **15**:261–275.

7. McKay RG *et al.*: **LV remodelling following myocardial infarction: a corollary to infarct expansion.** *Circulation* 1986, **74**:693–702.

8. Francis GS, McDonald KM: **LV hypertrophy: an initial response to myocardial injury.** *Am J Cardiol* 1992, **69** (Suppl G):3–9.

9. Anversa P *et al.*: **Cellular basis of ventricular remodelling after myocardial infarction.** *Am J Cardiol* 1991, **68**:7D–16D.

10. Rossi MA, Carillo SV: **Cardiac hypertrophy to pressure and volume overload: distinctly different biological phenomena?** *Int J Cardiol* 1991, **31**:133–142.

11. Capasso JM, Anversa P: **Mechanical performance of spared myocytes after myocardial infarction in rats, effects of captopril treatment.** *Am J Physiol* 1992, **263**:H841–H849.

12. Weber KT *et al.*: **Fibrillar collagen and remodelling of dilated canine left ventricle.** *Circulation* 1990, **82**:1387–1401.

13. Weber KT, Brilla CG: **Pathological hypertrophy and cardiac interstitium. Fibrosis and the renin angiotensin system.** *Circulation* 1991, **83**:1845–1865.

14. Treasure CB *et al.*: **Endothelium dependent dilation of the coronary microvasculature is impaired in dilated cardiomyopathy.** *Circulation* 1991, **81**:772–779.

15. Picard MH *et al.*: **Long-term effects of acute thrombolytic therapy on ventricular size and function.** *Am Heart J* 1993, **126**:1–10.

16. Nidorf SM *et al.*: **Benefit of late coronary reperfusion on ventricular morphology and function after myocardial infarction.** *J Am Coll Cardiol* 1993, **21**:683–691.

17. Meijer A *et al.*: **LV function after successful coronary thrombolysis: impact of reocclusion.** *J Am Coll Cardiol* 1994, **23**:129A [Abstract].

18. Jeremy RW *et al.*: **Infarct artery perfusion and changes in LV volume in the month after myocardial infarction.** *J Am Coll Cardiol* 1987, **9**:989–995.

19. Connelly CM *et al.*: **Effects of reperfusion after coronary occlusion on post-infarct scar tissue.** *Circ Res* 1985, **57**:562–577.

20. Marban E: **Myocardial stunning and hibernation: the physiology behind the colloquialisms.** *Circulation* 1991, **83**:681–688.

21. Gwilt DJ *et al.*: **Myocardial infarct size and mortality in diabetic patients.** *Br Heart J* 1985, **54**:466–472.

22. Gaudron P *et al.*: **Progressive LV dysfunction and remodelling after myocardial infarction.** *Circulation* 1993, **87**:755–763.

23. Lamas GA *et al.*: **Effects of LV shape and captopril therapy on exercise capacity after anterior wall acute myocardial infarction.** *Am J Cardiol* 1989, **63**:135–141.

24. White HD *et al.*: **LV end-systolic volume as the major determinant of survival after recovery from myocardial infarction.** *Circulation* 1987, **76**:44–51.

25. Pasternack RC *et al.*: **Acute myocardial infarction.** In *Heart Disease*, 4th edn. Edited by E. Braunwald, Philadelphia: WB Saunders, 1992, pp1200–1291.

26. Ishihara H *et al.*: **Relation between ventriculoarterial coupling and myocardial energetics in patients with idiopathic dilated cardiomyopathy.** *J Am Coll Cardiol* 1994, **23**:406–416.

27. Muller AF *et al.*: **Regional blood flow in chronic heart failure: the reason for the lack of correlation between patients exercise tolerance and cardiac output?** *Br Heart J* 1992, **67**:478–481.

28. Motwani JG *et al.*: **Effectiveness of captopril in reversing renal vasoconstriction after Q-wave acute myocardial infarction.** *Am J Cardiol* 1993, **71**:281–286.

29. Harris P: **Congestive cardiac failure: central role of the arterial pressure.** *Br Heart J* 1987, **58**:190–203.

30. McAlpine HM *et al.*: **Neuroendocrine activation after acute myocardial infarction.** *Br Heart J* 1988, **60**:117–124.

31. Valori C *et al.*: **Free noradrenaline and adrenaline excretion in relation to clinical syndromes following myocardial infarction.** *Am J Cardiol* 1967, **20**:605–617.

32. Malliani A, Schwartz PJ: **A sympathetic reflex elicited by experimental coronary occlusion.** *Am J Physiol* 1969, **217**:703–709.

33. Staszewska-Barczak J: **The reflex stimulation of catecholamine secretion during the acute stage of myocardial infarction in the dog.** *Clin Sci* 1971, **41**:419–439.

34. Kjellgren O, Gomes JA: **Heart rate variability and baroreflex sensitivity in myocardial infarction.** *Am Heart J* 1993, **125**:204–215.

35. Farrell TG *et al.*: **Risk stratification for arrhythmic events in postinfarction patients based on heart rate variability, ambulatory electrocardiographic variables and the signal-averaged electrocardiogram.** *J Am Coll Cardiol* 1991, **18**:687–697.

36. Rouleau JL *et al.*: **Activation of neurohumoral systems in postinfarction LV dysfunction.** *J Am Coll Cardiol* 1993, **22**:390–398.

37. Davis JO, Freeman RH: **Mechanisms regulating renin release.** *Physiol Rev* 1976, **56**:1–56.

38. Ray SG *et al.*: **Circulating endothelin in acute ischaemia syndromes.** *Br Heart J* 1992, **67**:383–386.

39. Stewart DJ *et al.*: **Increased plasma endothelin-1 in the early hours of acute myocardial infarction.** *J Am Coll Cardiol* 1991, **18**:38–43.

40. Yasuda M *et al.*: **Circulating immunoreactive endothelin in ischaemic heart disease.** *Am Heart J* 1990, **119**:801–806.

41. Stewart DJ, Baffour R: **Functional state of the endothelium determines the response to endothelin in the coronary circulation.** *Cardiovasc Res* 1990, **24**:7–12.

42. Miyauchi T et al.: **Involvement of endothelin in the regulation of human vascular tonus.** Circulation 1990, 81:1874–1880.

43. McMurray JJ et al.: **Elevated plasma endothelin concentrations in chronic heart failure: evidence for renal clearance and failure to increase with exercise.** Circulation 1992, 85:1374–1379.

44. Fontana F et al.: **Plasma atrial natriuretic factor in patients with acute myocardial infarction.** Eur Heart J 1990, 11:779–787.

45. Tan AICTL et al.: **Atrial natriuretic peptide after acute myocardial infarction.** Am Heart J 1989, 118:490–494.

46. Morita E et al.: **Increased levels of brain natriuretic peptide in patients with acute myocardial infarction.** Circulation 1993, 88:82–91.

47. Sigurdsson A et al.: **Short- and long-term neurohormonal activation following acute myocardial infarction.** Am Heart J 1993, 126:1068–1076.

48. Yasue H et al.: **Increased secretion of atrial natriuretic polypeptide from the left ventricle in patients with dilated cardiomyopathy.** J Clin Invest 1989, 83:46–51.

49. Holmes SJ et al.: **Renal, endocrine and haemodynamic effects of human brain natriuretic peptide in normal man.** J Clin Endocrinol Metab 1993, 76:91–96.

50. Torstilla I: **The plasma kinin system in acute myocardial infarction.** Acta Med Scand 1978, (Suppl 620):1–78.

51. Rasmanis G et al.: **Prostacyclin production in myocardial infarction in the acute phase and during follow-up.** J Intern Med 1991, 229:135–141.

52. Francis GS et al.: **Comparison of neuroendocrine activation in patients with LV dysfunction with and without congestive heart failure.** Circulation 1990, 82:1724–1729.

53. Omland T et al.: **Prognostic value of atrial natriuretic factor, norepinephrine and epinephrine in acute myocardial infarction.** Am J Cardiol 1993, 72:255–259.

54. Pfeffer M et al.: **Effect of captopril on mortality and morbidity in patients with LV dysfunction after myocardial infarction.** N Engl J Med 1992, 327:669–677.

55.The SOLVD Investigators: **Effect of enalapril on mortality and the development of heart failure in asymptomatic patients with reduced LV ejection fractions.** N Engl J Med 1992, 327:685–691.

56. Jugdutt BI, Warnica JW: **Intravenous nitroglycerine therapy to limit myocardial infarct size, expansion and complications. Effect of timing, dose and infarct location.** Circulation 1988, 78:906–919.

57. GISSI 3: **Effects of lisinopril and transdermal glyceryl trinitrate singly and together on 6-week mortality and ventricular function after acute myocardial infarction.** Lancet 1994, 343:1115–1122.

58. ISIS Collaborative Group: **ISIS-4. Randomised study of oral captopril in over 50,000 patients with suspected acute myocardial infarction.** Circulation 1993, 88 (Suppl):394.

59. Sharpe N et al.: **Early prevention of LV dysfunction following myocardial infarction.** Lancet 1991, i:872–874.

60. Bonaduce D et al.: **Effects of captopril treatment on LV remodelling and function after anterior myocardial infarction: comparison with digitalis.** J Am Coll Cardiol 1992, 19:858–863.

61.Woods K et al.: **Intravenous magnesium sulphate in suspected acute myocardial infarction: results of the second Leicester Intravenous Magnesium Intervention Trial (LIMIT-2).** Lancet 1992, 339:1553–1558.

62. Goldstein RE et al.: **The Adverse Experience Committee; and the Multicenter Diltiazem Post-infarction Research Group.** Circulation 1991, 83:52–60.

63. Goldbourt U et al. for the SPRINT Study Group: **Early administration of nifedipine in suspected acute myocardial infarction. The Secondary Prevention Reinfarction Israel Nifedipine Trial 2 Study.** Arch Intern Med 1993, 153:345–353.

64. Held P: **Effects of beta blockers on ventricular dysfunction after myocardial infarction: tolerability and survival effects.** Am J Cardiol 1993, 71:39C–44C.

65. Waagstein F et al.: **Beneficial effects of metoprolol in idiopathic dilated cardiomyopathy.** Lancet 1993, 342:1441–1446.

66. Elefteriades JA et al.: **Coronary artery bypass grafting in severe LV dysfunction: excellent survival with improved ejection fraction and functional state.** J Am Coll Cardiol 1993, 22:1411–1417.

67. Ray SG et al.: **Captopril after acute myocardial infarction.** Br Heart J 1993, 69:215–222.

68. St John Sutton M et al.: **Quantitative two-dimensional echocardiographic measurements are major predictors of adverse cardiovascular events after acute myocardial infarction.** Circulation 1994, 89:68–75.

69. Sharpe N et al.: **Treatment of patients with symptomless LV dysfunction after myocardial infarction.** Lancet 1988, i:255–259.

70. Bonarjee W et al.: **Attenuation of LV dilatation after acute myocardial infarction by early initiation of enalapril therapy.** Am J Cardiol 1993, 72:1004–1009.

71. Bazzino O et al.: **Early treatment with low dose enalapril prevents LV dilatation after acute myocardial infarction.** Circulation 1992, 86 (Suppl I):I454.

72. Konstam MA et al.: **Effects of the angiotensin converting enzyme inhibitor enalapril on the long-term progression of LV dysfunction in patients with heart failure.** Circulation 1992, 86:431–438.

73. Konstam MA et al. for the SOLVD Investigators: **Effects of the angiotensin converting enzyme inhibitor enalapril on the long-term progression of LV dilatation in patients with asymptomatic systolic dysfunction.** Circulation 1993, 88:2277–2283.

74. Greenberg B et al.: **Effects of long-term enalapril therapy on echocardiographic variables in SOLVD patients.** Circulation 1992, 86 (Suppl): I251 [abstract].

75. Cleland JGF: **ACE inhibitors for the prevention and treatment of heart failure: insights from the SOLVD trials.** Eur Heart J 1994, 15:125–130.

76. Dahlöf B et al.: **Reversal of LV hypertrophy in hypertensive patients: a metaanalysis of 109 treatment studies.** Am J Hypertens 1992, 5:95–110.

77. Weber KT et al.: **Myocardial fibrosis: functional significance and regulatory factors.** Cardiovasc Res 1993, 27:341–348.

78. Weber KT, Brilla CG: **Pathological hypertrophy and cardiac interstitium. Fibrosis and renin-angiotensin aldosterone system.** Circulation 1991, 83:1849–1865.

79. Pouleur HG et al.: **Changes in ventricular volume, wall thickness and wall stress during progression of LV dysfunction.** Am J Cardiol 1993, 22 (Suppl):43A–48A.

80. Gotzsche CO et al.: **Effects of captopril on LV systolic and diastolic function after acute myocardial infarction.** Am J Cardiol 1992, 70:156–160.

81. Zelis R et al.: A comparison of the effects of vasodilator stimuli on peripheral resistance vessels in normal subjects and in patients with congestive heart failure. J Clin Invest 1968, 47:960–970.

82. Puri S et al.: Increased alveolar-capillary membrane resistance to gas transfer in patients with chronic heart failure. Br Heart J 1994, 72:40–44.

83. Cleland JGF et al.: The effects of frusemide and angiotensin-converting enzyme inhibitors and their combination on cardiac and renal haemodynamics in heart failure. Eur Heart J 1988, 9:132–141.

84. Cleland JGF et al.: Effects of enalapril in heart failure: a double blind study of effects on exercise performance, renal function, hormones, and metabolic state. Br Heart J 1985, 54:305–312.

85. Cleland JGF et al.: Captopril in heart failure: a double blind controlled trial. Br Heart J 1984, 52:530–535.

86. Webster MW et al.: Effects of enalapril on ventricular arrhythmias in heart failure. Am J Cardiol 1985, 56:566.

87. Fletcher R D et al.: Enalapril decreases prevalence of ventricular tachycardia in patients with chronic congestive heart failure. Circulation 1993, 87 (Suppl VI):VI49–VI56.

88. Packer M et al.: Effect of captopril on ventricular arrhythmias and sudden death in patients with LV dysfunction after myocardial infarction: SAVE trial. J Am Coll Cardiol 1993, 21 (Suppl):130A [abstract].

89. Pratt C et al. for the SOLVD Investigators: Lack of long-term ventricular arrhythmia reduction by enalapril in heart failure patients: double-blind, parallel, placebo controlled trial. Circulation 1991, 84 (Suppl II):II348.

90. Cleland JGF: ACE inhibition and heart failure: arrhythmias, catecholamines and electrolytes. Cardiologia 1990, 35 (Suppl 1):441–447.

91. Bashir Y et al.: Comparative electrophysiological effects of captopril or hydralazine combined with nitrate in patients with LV dysfunction and inducible ventricular tachycardia. Br Heart J 1992, 67:355–360.

92. Yusuf S et al.: Effect of enalapril on myocardial infarction and unstable angina in patients with low ejection fractions. Lancet 1992, 340:1173–1178.

93. Ball SG et al.: ACE inhibition, atherosclerosis and myocardial infarction — The AIRE study in practice. Eur Heart J 1994, 15 (Suppl B):20–25.

94. Cohn JN et al.: A comparison of enalapril with hydralazine-isosorbide dinitrate in the treatment of chronic congestive heart failure. N Engl J Med 1991, 325:303–310.

95. Captopril Multi-Center Research Group: A placebo-controlled trial of captopril in refractory chronic congestive heart failure. J Am Coll Cardiol 1983, 2:755–763.

96. Newman TJ et al.: Effects of captopril on survival in patients with heart failure. Am J Med 1988 84 (Suppl 3A):140–143.

97. Fonarow GC et al.: Effect of direct vasodilation with hydralazine versus angiotensin converting enzyme inhibition with captopril on mortality in advanced heart failure: The Hy-C Trial. Am J Cardiol 1992, 19:842–850.

98. The CONSENSUS Trial Study Group: Effects of enalapril on mortality in severe congestive heart failure. Results of the Cooperative North Scandinavian Enalapril Survival Study (CONSENSUS). N Engl J Med 1987, 316:1429–1435.

99. The SOLVD Investigators: Effect of enalapril on survival in patients with reduced LV ejection fractions and congestive heart failure. N Engl J Med 1991, 325:293–302.

100. Cleland JGF, Puri S: How do ACE inhibitors reduce mortality in patients with LV dysfunction with and without heart failure: remodelling, resetting or sudden death? Br Heart J 1994, 72 (Suppl 5):81–86.

CHAPTER 2

Risk stratification after myocardial infarction

John JV McMurray

Introduction

The purpose of risk stratification

The purpose of risk stratification following MI is to identify those patients with the greatest chance of a further adverse event, such as recurrent MI, chronic heart failure (CHF), arrhythmia or death. Such an exercise would, of course, be relatively futile unless it was considered that high-risk patients identified by such a process could be treated in a way that would improve their prognosis. In other words, risk stratification, as a concept, goes hand in hand with that of secondary prevention.

Risk stratification as the basis of secondary prevention

Implicit in the concept of risk stratification is that risk factors for adverse outcome are modifiable even though some major ones such as age and sex are not (*see* Figure 2.1). Risk factors are also often equated with pathophysiological mechanisms, implying cause and effect. In this way they are linked to specific, or targeted, pharmacological or other therapies. It is hoped that favourable modification of the risk factor by its specific treatment will lead to a reduction in a specific adverse outcome. Whether such a line of reasoning is correct is debatable. Ventricular arrhythmias would seem to be an obvious risk factor for sudden death and are statistically associated with that outcome. They also, however, identify patients at high risk of CHF. Specific anti-arrhythmic therapy may actually increase the risk of sudden death and total mortality, as in the CAST study [1]. ACE inhibitors, specifically targeted at ventricular dysfunction and reducing the risk of CHF, also reduce the risk of arrhythmias, sudden death and recurrent MI. The interaction between different risk factors, and even that between individual risk factors and treatments, is therefore complex and sometimes unpredictable.

Special investigations

If we accept that there are high-risk post-MI patients who can be identified and who will benefit from special treatment, how can we find them? Are special investigations necessary? Do they offer any additional information over that obtainable from the history, examination, 12-lead electrocardiogram (ECG), chest radiogram and simple biochemical tests that are usually carried out in most patients admitted with AMI? If so, which is the most predictive, safe and cost-effective? The remainder of this chapter will address these questions.

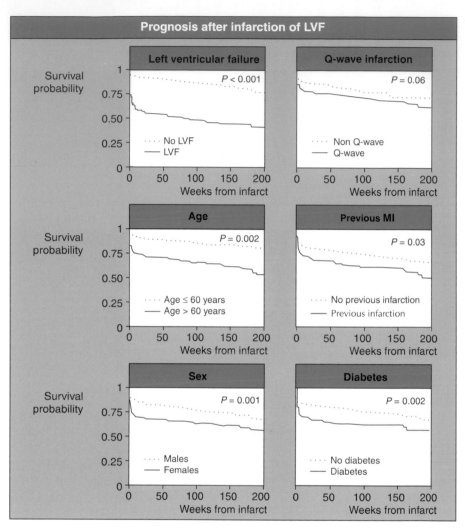

Figure 2.1. Kaplan–Meier survival curves illustrating the effects on prognosis after infarction of left ventricular failure (LVF), Q-wave infarction, age, sex, diabetes and history of myocardial infarction (MI). Adapted with permission from [2].

Ventricular dysfunction, heart failure and prognosis

Significance of clinical and radiological LV failure

A clinical diagnosis of LV failure (LVF) or diuretic prescription made during the in-hospital phase of AMI identifies patients with a poor short- and long-term prognosis (*see* Figure 2.1) [2].

Patients with radiological pulmonary congestion (PC)—about half of those with clinical LVF—are at even higher risk. Two-year mortality in patients without radiological PC in an analysis of MPIP combined with the placebo arm of MDPIT was 8.3%. In patients with mild, moderate or severe pulmonary congestion, two-year mortality was 15.2, 24.4 and 47.6%, respectively [3,4].

The combination of even transient signs of LVF, that is, any one of a third heart sound, persistent tachycardia or pulmonary crackles, or radiological pulmonary oedema, has been used to identify patients who are at high risk, and who would especially benefit from long-term treatment with an ACE inhibitor [5].

Is there incremental prognostic information from measurement of LV function?

Patients with early clinical or radiological LVF and impaired LV function have a particularly bad prognosis (*see* Table 2.1 and Figure 2.2). The risk of death is eight times that of patients without these risk factors [3,4]. However, even patients who have not manifested clinical or radiological LVF, but who do have impaired LV function, are at high risk (*see* Table 2.1). This is a large and important group of patients. Between 35 and 45% of MI survivors have a radionuclide LVEF below 0.40 [2,3]. Approximately two-thirds of these will not show radiological signs of LVF and 30–40% will not manifest clinical signs of LVF [3,4].

Table 2.1. Inter-relationship between left ventricular ejection fraction (LVEF) and pulmonary congestion in 790 MPIP and 1060 MDPIT patients. PC, (radiological) pulmonary congestion.

Inter-relationship between LVEF and pulmonary congestion		
	Proportion of patients (%)	2-year mortality (%)
LVEF ≤ 40%		
With PC	42	28
Without PC	58	18
LVEF > 40%		
With PC	16	13
Without PC	84	5

To date it has not been possible to predict LVEF accurately from simple clinical criteria (*see* Figure 2.3) [6]. Consequently special investigation is needed to identify a high-risk subgroup of post-MI patients, such as those with silent LV dysfunction. This is because randomized clinical trials have shown that such patients benefit from treatment with ACE inhibitors and, probably, beta blockers [7].

Which measure of LV function gives most prognostic information?

LV end-systolic volume (ESV) gives more prognostic information than LVEF in patients with a reduced LVEF (*see* Figure 2.4) [8]. ESV has, however, not been used as the criterion for randomizing patients to trials with clinical endpoints but LVEF has.

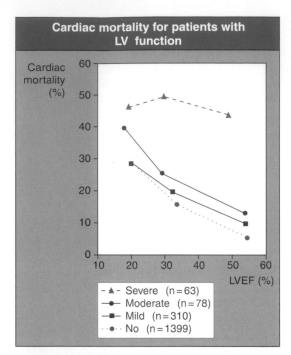

Cardiac mortality for patients with LV function

Figure 2.2. Cardiac mortality rate at three levels of predischarge left ventricular ejection fraction (LVEF) (<25%, 25 to 39% and ≥40%) and at four grades of pulmonary congestion (no, mild, moderate and severe). Each point represents mortality rate and mean LVEF in that combined category. Adapted with permission from [3].

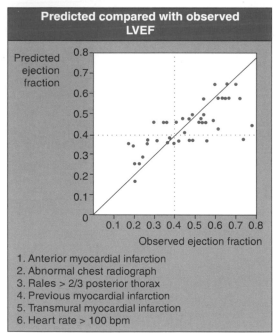

Predicted compared with observed LVEF

Figure 2.3. Six clinical variables most predictive of radionuclide left ventricular ejection fraction (LVEF) were selected by stepwise linear regression analysis. This model was then used to calculate a predicted ejection fraction for each patient and the predicted value was compared with the observed value. Even the optimal predictive model frequently failed to predict accurately the observed ejection fraction in individual cases. bpm, beats per minute. Adapted with permission from [6].

1. Anterior myocardial infarction
2. Abnormal chest radiograph
3. Rales > 2/3 posterior thorax
4. Previous myocardial infarction
5. Transmural myocardial infarction
6. Heart rate > 100 bpm

Figure 2.4. Actuarial curves for three groups of ejection fraction measurements, each subdivided according to whether end-systolic volume (ESV) was above or below the median for that group (the predictive value for ESV is apparent only when left ventricular ejection fraction [LVEF] is below 50%). Adapted with permission from [8].

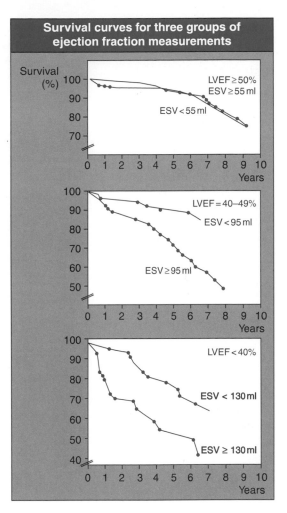

Which method should be used to measure LV function?

In most studies to date LV function has been measured by radionuclide ventriculography (RNVG). More recently echocardiography has become widely used in the CCU. Echocardiographic measurement of regional and global LV function has been found to be predictive of outcome. Echocardiography has been compared with RNVG and seems to give equal prognostic information, though the absolute LVEF measured by each method may be different [9].

LV function on exercise

The response of radionuclide (and echocardiographic) LV function to exercise has also been studied as a method of assessing risk post-MI. Usually resting LV function has been near normal in the patients in these studies. Failure of LVEF to increase, or a decrease in LVEF (especially if by more than 5%), identifies patients at increased risk of adverse outcome. Change in LVEF with exercise may give more prognostic information than ST segment change or reversible thallium perfusion defects in patients after MI [10].

Other measures of LV function

Stroke distance measured by Doppler ultrasound and systolic time intervals have been shown to give prognostic information post-MI, although their value with respect to other measures of LV function is unknown [11]. Plasma concentrations of the cardiac natriuretic peptides are also increased in patients with LV dysfunction post-MI. These markers are predictive of clinical outcome and elevated concentrations can be reduced by ACE inhibitor treatment. In future these peptides could be used as an alternative to echocardiography to choose patients for treatment and monitor the effects of treatment [12].

Myocardial ischaemia and risk of reinfarction

Resting 12-lead ECG

Non-Q-wave MI

Three large studies have consistently shown a higher incidence of in-hospital post-infarct angina in patients with non-Q-wave MI (average 45%) compared with those with Q-wave MI (average 23%) [13]. In these patients, angina associated with ST-T wave change is associated with a four-fold increase in risk of reinfarction and an approximate ten-fold increase in the risk of death at two weeks (11.5% compared with 1.5%). Patients with ST segment depression persisting at discharge have a one-year mortality of 22% compared with 5.5% in those without ST depression.

Pooled data from 14 studies reporting on nearly 5300 patients show that the increase of reinfarction between one week and three years post-MI is more than twice as high after non-Q-wave MI (16%) than after Q-wave MI (6%). Overall prognosis after non-Q wave MI is, however, better than after Q-wave MI (see Figure 2.1).

Non-Q-wave MI clearly identifies a group at very high risk of recurrent ischaemia/infarction. Furthermore, placebo-controlled randomized trials have shown that aspirin and diltiazem (but possibly not beta blockers) each reduce this risk by about half [13]. Routine coronary angiography and revascularization have been recommended for these patients, but there is no definite evidence of a prognostic benefit from this approach.

Recurrent ST segment change

The importance of transient ST segment elevation or depression (>1mm) and/or T-wave inversion occurring more than 24 hours from the onset of symptoms and before discharge was investigated in a GISSI substudy [14]. These changes were seen in 8% of patients, 86% of whom had Q-wave MI. In-hospital death, reinfarction and urgent revascularization occurred in 43% of patients with early ischaemia compared with 4.5% of the remaining patients. Survival without reinfarction remained significantly better in the patients without early ischaemia during six months of follow-up.

Angina pectoris

In clinical trials angina has been reported in 8–12% of post-MI patients at the time of discharge. The presence of angina is associated with an up to ten-fold increase in the risk of early reinfarction and death [15–17]. In patients with early post-MI angina, first-year mortality was 15% compared with 3% in those without. Early post-MI angina also appears to predict late adverse outcome. The exercise ECG appears to add no prognostic information in these patients. Indeed, early post-MI angina may be a better predictor of death than coronary angiography [15–17].

Angina occurring after discharge is recorded in approximately one-third of patients and seems to be a strong predictor of reinfarction (it may be the most powerful predictor). The one-year risk of reinfarction in patients with post-discharge angina is 8.6% compared with 3.9% in those without. Between 55 and 60% of patients who go on to develop fatal or non-fatal reinfarction are reported to have angina pectoris compared with 27% of event-free survivors [15–17].

Exercise ECG

Numerous studies have evaluated the role of the exercise ECG in predicting adverse outcome with conflicting results [18]. This reflects, at least in part, study size, patient selection, site of infarct, timing of the test post-MI, protocol used (submaximal compared with symptom limited), current medication and definition of adverse outcome (natural compared with physician-determined events, e.g. revascularization). The introduction of thrombolytic therapy may also have changed the predictive accuracy of the exercise ECG.

Patient selection may be particularly important in removing those at highest risk, either by carrying out early revascularization or by designating the patient unfit to exercise (e.g., because of age, CHF, or peripheral vascular disease). It is clear, however, that patients who can undertake an exercise ECG have a better prognosis than those who cannot. In the Multicenter Post Infarction Study the overall one-year mortality was 7.5%: 5% in patients able to perform a low-level exercise test, 17% in patients unable to exercise [19].

Up to half of symptom-limited post-MI exercise ECGs are positive, that is, are associated with ST segment change, poor exercise tolerance or the development of

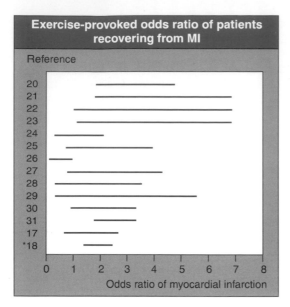

Figure 2.5. Exercise-provoked ST segment depression odds ratio with 95% confidence interval in patients recovering from recent myocardial infarction. y axis: numbers indicate reference numbers. *Meta-analysis. Adapted with permission from [18].

angina (a smaller proportion of submaximal tests are positive). The development of more than 1mm ST segment depression probably doubles the risk of an adverse event in the subsequent year (*see* Figure 2.5). ST segment depression may be more predictive in patients with inferior or non-Q-wave MI than in patients with anterior Q-wave MI. The combination of a poor exercise time (<6 minutes of the modified Bruce Protocol or <7 metabolic equivalents [METs]) and ST segment depression is a better predictor. With this combination the risk of reinfarction and death is increased three-fold (*see* Table 2.2) [32]. Even with these criteria, however, the positive predictive accuracy of exercise testing is low (<30%) and only a small proportion of total adverse events (perhaps about 5%) will occur in this very high-risk subgroup. The negative predictive accuracy, however, is high (up to 95%). Patients who manage a good exercise time and who do not develop ST segment depression have a very good prognosis (one-year mortality <2%).

The exercise test still seems to provide prognostic information in patients taking medication, including beta blockers, at the time of the test [33]. ST segment depression during concomitant ambulatory ECG monitoring may improve the predictive accuracy of the exercise ECG [34].

Ambulatory ECG

Both symptomatic and asymptomatic ST segment depression detected on the exercise ECG and ambulatory ECG identify patients at increased risk of reinfarction and death. The positive predictive value of such depression on ambulatory monitoring is low (<30%) and similar to that of ST segment depression on the exercise ECG. One report, however, suggests that ST segment depression during both types of test may be of more prognostic value (positive predictive value 63%) [34].

Interactions between relevant components of the exercise tolerance test and of stress thallium scintigraphy				
	Exercise duration (min)			Interaction *P*†
Exercise tolerance test	< 6	6.9	> 9	
ST depression ≥ 0.1 mV (1.0 mm)	Hazard ratio*			
Yes	3.4	1.9	1.1	< 0.01
No	0.8	0.9	1.0	
	Lung uptake			
Stress thallium scintigraphy	Increased	Not increased		
Reversible defect				
Yes	2.8	1.2		< 0.05
No	0.9	1.0		

Table 2.2. Interactions between relevant components of the exercise tolerance test and of stress thallium scintigraphy for the primary endpoint. *Ratio of the risk of primary endpoint events per unit of time among patients with the variable of interest to that among patients with the reference variable (unity value); †significance level for the lack of proportionality between the rows of hazard ratios. Reproduced with permission from [32].

Myocardial radionuclide perfusion imaging

A number of studies have examined the value of exercise stress thallium scanning as a means of determining risk post-MI. It is not clear whether thallium scanning adds any incremental prognostic information over a symptom-limited exercise ECG test. Some incremental prognostic information may be obtained from increased lung uptake of thallium, as this probably reflects impairment of LV function (*see* Table 2.2) [32]. However, exercise RNVG may still give more prognostic information than exercise thallium scanning.

Pharmacological stress thallium scintigraphy is a more recent approach to risk stratification; its value, however, remains to be defined.

Coronary angiography

Approximately 10% of survivors of MI have left main coronary artery stenosis and 30–40% have triple-vessel disease, that is, patterns of coronary artery disease for which coronary artery bypass surgery may improve survival. These patients tend to be older and their MI is more likely to be complicated by LVF, ventricular arrhythmias or post-infarct angina. They are also more likely to have had a previous MI.

A number of studies have shown that the coronary score adds little, if any, further prognostic information to that obtained from LV function [35]. Studies of routine compared with selective coronary angiography after thrombolytic therapy for MI have also been carried out. The consequent higher rate of revascularization in the routine groups did not lead to an improvement in short-term prognosis. In two post-MI studies where patients were randomized to medical or surgical treatment, survival was similar in each treatment group [35,36]. The major survival benefit of coronary artery bypass grafts (CABGs) may be confined to those with severe coronary disease and angina [11,35].

Electrical instability, ventricular arrhythmias and sudden death

Ambulatory ECG monitoring

Several large post-MI studies have shown that the 15–20% of patients who have more than ten ventricular ectopic beats (VEBs) per hour over 24 hours during ambulatory ECG monitoring, carried out more than 48 hours after MI, have a two- to four-fold increase in the risk of sudden death and overall mortality in the subsequent 1–3 years [19,37]. This association is even stronger for more complex arrhythmias (e.g. couplets, non-sustained ventricular tachycardia). Even with more complex arrhythmias, however, the positive predictive accuracy is only 5–38%, that is, only 4–7% of these patients go on to have an arrhythmic death in the next 1–2 years. Most patients who have frequent VEBs or more complex arrhythmias on ambulatory monitoring also have significantly impaired LV function. The combination of impaired LV function and ventricular arrhythmias increases the risk of sudden and total death 10–20-fold.

Ventricular dysfunction is a more powerful prognostic marker than are ventricular arrhythmias, and there is some debate in the literature as to whether ventricular arrhythmias give additional, independent, prognostic information.

Signal-averaged ECG

Low-amplitude late depolarizations (late potentials) at the end of the QRS complex may reflect a substrate for ventricular re-entry tachycardia and hence predict the likelihood of arrhythmic events [38]. Late potentials can be detected in the surface ECG using the techniques of high-gain amplification, low- and high-pass filtering and signal averaging. The highest frequency of late potentials is between seven and ten days post-MI when they may be present in up to 50% of patients (more in inferior MI), although this does depend on definition. The presence of late potentials increases the risk of an arrhythmic event (sustained ventricular tachycardia or sudden death) by up to nine-fold. However, the positive predictive accuracy of late potentials for an arrhythmic event is only 8–33% (higher for anterior than inferior MI), whereas the negative predictive accuracy is 96–99%. Late potentials do seem to be an independent predictor of arrhythmic events and may be a more powerful predictor of these events than LV function. The combination of the signal-averaged ECG (SAECG) with other investigations improves the prediction of adverse outcome. Interestingly, late potentials on an early SAECG also appear to predict the development of LV dilatation post-MI [39].

Autonomic function tests

More recently tests of autonomic function have been used to identify patients at increased risk of adverse outcome post-MI. Relatively little information on the value of these tests exists and their place in risk assessment has yet to be defined [40].

Heart rate variability

Altered autonomic activity in the form of an imbalance between the parasympathetic nervous system (PNS) and the SNS may be prognostically important post-MI [40]. Reduced heart rate variation, reflecting PNS activity, is associated with an up to seven-fold increase in the risk of arrhythmic events and death. Indeed, HRV seems to be the most accurate predictor of arrhythmic events when compared with LVEF, SAECG and clinical class. Positive predictive accuracy, however, is low (20%). Even when combined with the SAECG positive predictive accuracy increases to only 33%.

Baroreflex sensitivity

Injection of the pressor agent phenylephrine is normally associated with a baroreceptor-mediated reflex bradycardia; baroreflex sensitivity (BRS) reflects the relationship of the change in systolic blood pressure to the change in RR interval in the ECG. Patients with BRS are more prone to arrhythmic events. In one study depressed BRS was associated with a 36-fold increase in the risk of an arrhythmic event [40]. The St George's group has reported the positive accuracy of depressed BRS to be 44–64%. When compared with other investigations, depressed BRS has so far been found to be the most accurate independent predictor of sudden death and ventricular arrhythmias. BRS has been reported to be superior to reduced HRV, 24-hour ECG VEBs, and SAECG and exercise ECG, even in combination. Interestingly, BRS does not appear to correlate with LVEF or late potentials on the SAECG.

Programmed electrical stimulation

In a recent study, routine testing of over 1200 MI survivors by programmed electrical stimulation (PES) yielded a positive result in approximately 6% of patients [41]. Fewer than 20% of these patients went on to sustain an arrhythmic event (i.e., about 1% of all tested patients), which was fatal in fewer than 40% of cases.

Even in high-risk patients the positive predictive accuracy of PES is only about 30%. Other, non-invasive, tests give the same or better prognostic information. For example, a patient with a low LVEF and late potentials has a 25% risk of an arrhythmic event in the first year post-MI. In patients with normal LV function the very low risk of an arrhythmic event argues against any consideration of PES. Similarly, the high negative predictive accuracy of the SAECG argues against further investigation even of patients with a positive SAECG with a low LVEF who do not have late potentials. Even in these patients there must be doubts about the value of PES.

The ESVEM study has not shown PES to be a better method of choosing therapy than the ambulatory and exercise ECG [42]. Most importantly of all, however, CAST has raised doubts about the value of anti-arrhythmic therapy at all, especially with class I agents [1].

Interrelation of risk factors

It is clear that attempting to separate risk factors is artificial. For example, patients with poor LV function are not only most likely to develop heart failure, but they are also at high risk of recurrent MI and ventricular arrhythmias. For this reason the summation of risk factors does not give an ideal refinement of prognosis (*see* Figure 2.6) [19].

For the same reason sequential, multiple, investigations add relatively little incremental information (*see* Figure 2.7) [8]. Nevertheless, small, very high-risk, subgroups can be identified.

Clinical risk stratification scoring systems

Several studies have compared the usefulness of data obtained from special investigations with that obtained from clinical examination and routine tests at the time

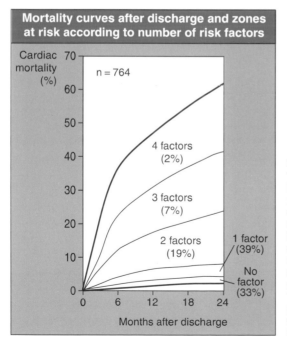

Figure 2.6. The risk factors were New York Heart Association functional class II to IV before admission, pulmonary rales, occurrence of ten or more ventricular ectopic depolarizations per hour, and a radionuclide ejection fraction below 0.40. The variation of risk within each zone reflects the spectrum of relative risk for individual factors as well as the range of mulitiplicative risks for combinations of two and three factors. The numbers in parentheses denote the percentage of the population with the specified number of factors. Adapted with permission from [19].

Figure 2.7. Combination of post-myocardial infarction (MI) investigations giving the highest probability of severe complications (severe angina, severe heart failure, reinfarction, angioplasty, cardiac surgery or death). ExT, conventional exercise test; T1, thallium-201 scintigraphy; Echo, echocardiograph; RNVG, radionuclide ventriculography; C, cardiac catheterization. Adapted with permission from [19].

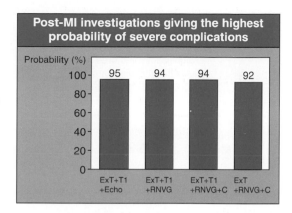

of MI (e.g. chest radiogram, 12-lead ECG) [43–45]. Special investigation seems to add little additional predictive information. This is probably because several major risk factors are clinical variables, such as previous MI, age and sex. Symptomatic LV dysfunction and angina are also important risk factors. It seems that most further incremental information may be obtained only from measurement of LV function.

Which test is best?

It seems clear that the single variable that best predicts prognosis after MI is LV function. LV function can be measured accurately, objectively, reproducibly, non-invasively and cheaply. The subgroup of patients with poor LV function (i.e. LVEF < 40%) also contains many of those with prognostically significant coronary artery disease (i.e. who might benefit from surgery) and most of those with prognostically important ventricular arrhythmias. Not only does measurement of LV function risk stratify patients, but it also identifies those who will benefit from a particular pharmacological intervention or interventions (i.e., an ACE inhibitor and, probably, beta blocker). Thus, measurement of LV function fulfils the main objective of risk stratification post-MI, that is, the identification of high-risk patients who will benefit from secondary prevention. As yet it is not clear that any other test definitely fulfils both these requirements. It is possible that coronary artery bypass surgery improves survival in patients with certain patterns of coronary artery disease and easily inducible ischaemia, even if this is painless. For this reason some form of stress test to detect reversible ischaemia may also be routinely indicated in MI survivors (*see* Figure 2.7). The test used will depend on local expertise, the patient's ability to exercise and how abnormal the baseline ECG is. The main value of the exercise test is, however, the high negative predictive value of a negative test.

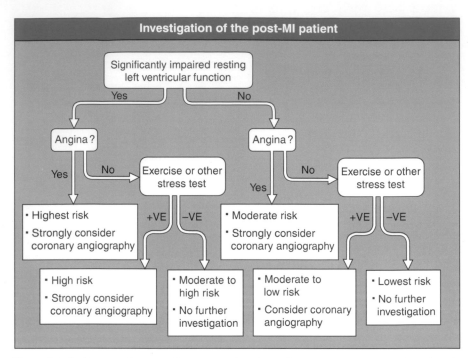

Figure 2.8. Positive exercise test indicates more than 1 mm ST segment depression at less than six minutes on modified Bruce. +ve, positive; -ve, negative.

The algorithm in Figure 2.8 deliberately does not attempt to evaluate electrical instability. This is partly because it is still not certain whether ambulatory ECG monitoring gives significant incremental information, and because the role of other electrical investigations has yet to be fully defined. Most importantly, however, the algorithm does not routinely advocate such tests because it remains to be proved that there is a specific secondary prevention therapy that will reduce the likelihood of a significant arrhythmia and improve prognosis. Class Ic anti-arrhythmic drugs have manifestly failed in this respect. Amiodarone looks more promising but more randomized clinical trials are awaited.

References

1. The Cardiac Arrhythmia Suppression Trial II Investigators: Effect of the antiarrhythmic agent moricizine on survival after myocardial infarction. *N Engl J Med* 1992, **327**:227–233.

2. Stevenson R *et al.*: Short and long term prognosis in acute myocardial infarction since introduction of thrombolysis. *BMJ* 1993, **307**:349–353.

3. Gottlieb S *et al.*: Interrelation of LV ejection fraction, pulmonary congestion and outcome in acute myocardial infarction. *Am J Cardiol* 1992, **69**:977–984.

4. Nicod P *et al.*: Influence on prognosis and morbidity of LV ejection fraction with and without signs of LV failure after acute myocardial infarction. *Am J Cardiol* 1988, **61**:1651–1171.

5. The AIRE Study Investigators: Effect of ramipril on mortality and morbidity of survivors of acute myocardial infarction with clinical evidence of heart failure. *Lancet* 1993, **342**:821–828.

6. Sanford CF *et al.*: Value of radionuclide ventriculography

in the immediate characterization of patients with acute myocardial infarction. *Am J Cardiol* 1982, **49**:637–644.

7. Pfeffer MA *et al.*: **Effect of captopril on mortality and morbidity in patients with LV dysfunction after myocardial infarction.** *N Engl J Med* 1992, **327**:6679–6687.

8. White HD *et al.*: **LV end systolic volume as the major determinant of survival after recovery from myocardial infarction.** *Circulation* 1987, **76**:4451.

9. Candell-Riera J *et al.*: **Uncomplicated first myocardal infarction: strategy for comprehensive prognostic studies.** *J Am Coll Cardiol* 1991, **18**:1207–1219.

10. Roig E *et al.*: **Prognostic value of exercise radionuclide angiography in low risk acute myocardial infarction survivors.** *Eur Heart J* 1993, **14**:213–218.

11. Northover B: **Impact on survival of a decade of change in the management of patients who have sustained a myocardial infarction.** *Cardiology* 1993, **83**:82–92.

12. Motwani JG *et al.*: **Plasma brain natriuretic peptide as an indicator for angiotensin converting enzyme inhibition after myocardial infarction.** *Lancet* 1993, **341**:1109–1113.

13. Gibson RS: **Non-Q-wave myocardial infarction: diagnosis, prognosis and management.** *Curr Probl Cardiol* 1988, **13**:9–72.

14. Silva P *et al.*: **Prognostic significance of early ischaemia after acute myocardial infarction in low risk patients.** *Am J Cardiol* 1993, **72**:1142–1147.

15. Gilpin E *et al.*: **Factors associated with recurrent myocardial infarction within one year after acute myocardial infarction.** *Am Heart J* 1991, **121**:457–465.

316. Galjee MA *et al.*: **The prognostic value, clinical and angiographic characteristics of patients with early post-infarction angina after a first myocardial infarction.** *Am Heart J* 1992, **125**:4855.

17. Jespersen CM *et al.*: **The prognostic significance of post-infarction angina pectoris and the effect of verapamil on the incidence of angina pectoris and prognosis.** *Eur Heart J* 1994, **15**:270–276.

18. Jespersen CM *et al.*: **Exercise-provoked ST-segment depression and prognosis in patients recovering from acute myocardial infarction. Significance and pitfalls.** *J Intern Med* 1993, **233**:2732.

19. The Multicenter Post Infarction Research Group: **Risk stratification and survival after myocardial infarction.** *N Engl J Med* 1983, **309**: 331–336.

20. Theroux P *et al.*: **Prognostic value of exercise testing soon after myocardial infarction.** *N Engl J Med* 1979, **301**:341–345.

21. Smith JW *et al.*: **Exercise testing three weeks after myocardial infarction.** *Chest* 1979, **75**:12–16.

22. Sami M: **The prognostic significance of serial exercise testing after myocardial infarction.** *Circulation* 1979, **60**:1238–1246.

23. Jespersen CM *et al.*: **The prognostic value of maximal exercise testing soon after the first myocardial infarction.** *Eur Heart J* 1985, **6**:769–772.

24. Handler CE: **Submaximal predischarge exercise testing after myocardial infarction: prognostic value and limitations.** *Eur Heart J* 1985, **6**:510–517.

25. Starling MR *et al.*: **Exercise testing early after myocardial infarction: predictive value for subsequent unstable angina and death.** *Am J Cardiol* 1980, **46**:909–914.

26. Williams WL *et al.*: **Comparison of clinical and treadmill variables for the prediction of outcome after myocardial infarction.** *J Am Coll Cardiol* 1984, **4**:477–486.

27. Jelinek VM *et al.*: **Assessment of cardiac risk 10 days after** uncomplicated myocardial infarction. *BMJ* 1982, **284**:227–230.

28. Sullivan ID *et al.*: **Submaximal exercise testing early after myocardial infarction. Prognostic importance of exercise induced ST segment elevation.** *Br Heart J* 1984, **52**:147–153.

29. Hung J *et al.*: **Comparative value of maximal treadmill testing, exercise myocardial perfusion scintigraphy and exercise radionuclide ventriculography for distinguishing high- and low-risk patients soon after acute myocardial infarction.** *Am J Cardiol* 1984, **53**:1221–1227.

30. Weld FM *et al.*: **Risk stratification with low-level exercise testing two weeks after acute myocardial infarction.** *Circulation* 1981, **64**:306–314.

31. Klein J *et al.*: **Does the rest electrocardiogram after myocardial infarction determine the predictive value of exercise-induced ST segment depression? A 2 year follow-up study in a veteran population.** *J Am Coll Cardiol* 1989, **14**:305–311.

32. Moss AJ *et al.*: **Detection and significance of myocardial ischaemia in stable patients after recovery from an acute coronary event.** *JAMA* 1993, **269**:2379–2385.

33. Lim R *et al.*: **Exercise testing without interruption of medication for refining the selection of mildly symptomatic patients for prognostic coronary angiography.** *Br Heart J* 1994, **71**:334–340.

34. Jereckek M *et al.*: **Prognostic value of ischaemia during Holter monitoring and exercise testing after acute myocardial infarction.** *Am J Cardiol* 1993, **72**:813.

35. Norris RM *et al.*: **Prognosis after recovery from myocardial infarction: the relative importance of cardiac dilatation and coronary stenoses.** *Eur Heart J* 1992, **13**:1611–1618.

36. Lorimer AR *et al.*: **The role of early surgery following myocardial infarction.** *Br J Clin Pract* 1992, **46**:238–242.

37. Bigger JT *et al.*: **The relationships among ventricular arrhythmias, LV dysfunction and mortality in the 2 years after myocardial infarction.** *Circulation* 1984, **69**:250–258.

38. Gomes JA *et al.*: **Post myocardial infarction stratification and the signal-averaged electrocardiogram.** *Prog Cardiovasc Dis* 1993, **35**:263–270.

39. Zaman AG *et al.*: **Late potentials and ventricular enlargement after myocardial infarction.** *Circulation* 1993, **88**:905–914.

40. Turner A *et al.*: **Autonomic function testing following myocardial infarction.** *Br J Hosp Med* 1994, **51**:89–96.

41. Bourke J *et al.*: **Routine programmed electrical stimulation in survivors of acute myocardial infarction for prediction of spontaneous ventricular tachyarrhythmias during follow-up: results, optimal stimulation protocol and cost-effective screening.** *J Am Coll Cardiol* 1991, **18**:780–788.

42. Mason JW for the ESVEM investigators: **A comparison of electrophysiological testing with Holter monitoring to predict antiarrhythmic drug therapy for ventricular tachyarrhythmias.** *N Engl J Med* 1993, **329**:445–451.

43. Myers MG *et al.*: **Are routine non-invasive tests useful in prediction of outcome after myocardial infarction in elderly people?** *Lancet* 1993, **342**:1069–1072.

44. Hillis LD, *et al.*: **Risk stratification before thrombolytic therapy in patients with acute myocardial infarction.** *J Am Coll Cardiol* 1990, **16**:313–315.

45. Arnold AER *et al.*: **Prediction of mortality following hospital discharge after thrombolysis for acute myocardial infarction: is there a need for coronary angiography?** *Eur Heart J* 1993, **14**:306–315.

CHAPTER 3

Overview of large clinical trials
in patients with myocardial infarction

John GF Cleland

Introduction

The major single factor influencing the management of MI has been the results of the "mega-trials". These were made possible by the development of CCUs which provided a focus for medical, nursing and technician expertise, and the study of large numbers of patients in a relatively homogeneous environment. While the "mega-trials" are useful sign-posts, interpretation needs to be tailored to the individual patient. Benefit in one subgroup may be offset by harm in another, while producing no apparent overall effect. Subset analysis within the "mega-trials" has become more accurate as the size of the trials has grown. Nevertheless, care must be taken when interpreting data. For example, it has been shown that lisinopril improves prognosis in most patients with MI over the first six weeks. It is unclear whether those patients who benefit can be identified prospectively. It is also unclear whether long-term treatment with an ACE inhibitor is warranted in all patients, although it certainly is in substantial subgroups. In addition, although analyses of trials according to the treatment they were allocated to, and not to the treatment they actually received, is the correct approach, it may underestimate the magnitude of the treatment's effect, whether the effect is harmful or beneficial.

It is also difficult to determine for how long treatment should be administered. If a treatment reduces mortality in one group it can be argued that, since that group contains more patients at high risk (i.e., whose lives have been saved), failure of the curves to come together may indicate continuing benefit from therapy and therefore that long-term treatment should be continued. This is only true if the treatment does not irrevocably change the substrate. Antibiotics for infection and thrombolysis for MI are two examples where the benefits of treatment often greatly outlast the duration of treatment.

General care of patients after myocardial infarction

A summary of studies of mortality following MI using various treatment modalities is shown in Table 3.1.

Hypoxia is common after MI, predicts a worse prognosis and can be readily detected by blood sampling or by transcutaneous oximetry. Whether this should be detected and treated is unproven. Hyperbaric oxygen is not generally available but an isolated clinical trial by Thurston *et al.* in 1973 suggested benefit [1]. However, a study by Rawles and Kenmure in 1976 suggested that unrestricted use of oxygen may have deleterious effects [2].

General care post-MI			
Intervention	No. of patients Follow-up	Comparisons	Mortality
Oxygen Thurston 1973 [1]	208 Hospital mortality (usually 3 weeks)	*Hyperbaric oxygen* Usual care	*16.5%* 22.9% RRR 28% *P* < 0.05
Oxygen Rawles 1976 [2]	157 Hospital mortality (definite MIs only)	*Oxygen* Air	*11.3%* 3.9% R.Excess R 290% *ns*
Mobile CCU Wennerblom 1982 [3]	821 Hospital mortality	*Mobile CCU* Standard ambulance	*17.2%* 32.8% RRR 48% *P* < 0.05
Mobile CCU Mathewson 1985 [4]	781 28-day mortality	*Mobile CCU* Standard ambulance	*50%* 63% RRR 21% *P* < 0.001
Diazepam Dixon 1980 [5}	131 48 hours	*Diazepam (10 mg daily)* Placebo	*1 death* *8 VTs or VFs* 3 deaths 8VTs or VFs

Table 3.1. MI, myocardial infarction; RRR, relative risk reduction; R.Excess R, relative excess risk; *ns*, non-significant; CCU, coronary care unit; VT, ventricular tachycardia; VF, ventricular fibrillation.

Pai *et al.* [6] found that the 28-day mortality from MI was still depressingly high at 36%, with 59% of deaths occurring before reaching hospital out of 1001 MIs occurring in the community. In the study, 56 patients had a cardiac arrest in the presence of the family practitioner, 21 were resuscitated and reached hospital, while 13 patients survived until discharge. Wennerblom *et al* [3] compared the effects of a mobile CCU with usual care on outcome of MIs in the community. The resuscitation rates were not higher than those of the family practitioners in the study by Pai, with only two of 36 patients having cardiac arrests surviving until hospital discharge. Although the only other possibly effective treatments available to the mobile units were opiates, nitrates, lignocaine and frusemide, patients so treated had a striking reduction in pre- and in-hospital mortality. The study of Mathewson *et al.* [4], pre-dating thrombolysis, also showed striking reductions in mortality with early care, presumably attributable to good analgesia, heart-failure treatment, atropine and defibrillation based in a mobile CCU.

The relatively small short-term study of Dixon *et al.* [5] failed to show a significant reduction in serious arrhythmias with diazepam. Anxiety rating was also no lower on diazepam but drowsiness and respiratory depression were more common. Rivers *et al.* [7] suggests that the rate of reinfarction in the first year after initial MI could be reduced from 12.5 to 6.3% merely by getting the patient to stop smoking.

Thrombolytic therapy after myocardial infarction

Selected major randomized controlled studies of thrombolysis after MI are given in Table 3.2.

Randomized, controlled studies of thrombolysis after MI				
Study Duration of pain	No. of patients Follow-up	Comparisons	Mortality (early)	Mortality (late)
GISSI-I [8,9] 1986 Open label entry: < 12 hours	11 712 Early: 21 days Late: 12 months	SK (1.5 MU) Unblinded control	10.7% 13.0% RRR 19% P=0.0002	17.2% 19.0% RRR 10% P=0.0008
ISIS-II [10] 1988 Double-blind entry: < 24 hours	17 187 Early: 5 weeks Late: 15 months	SK (1.5 MU) Placebo	9.2% 12.0% RRR 25% P<0.00001	17.8% 20.4% RRR 22% P<0.00001
AIMS [11] 1990 Double-blind entry: < 6 hours	1004 Early: 30 days Late: 12 months	APSAC (300 U) + IV Heparin Placebo + IV Heparin	6.4% 12.1% RRR 51% P=0.0006	11.1% 17.8% RRR 43% P=0.0007
ASSET [12,13] 1990 Double-blind entry: < 5 hours	2516 Early: 4 weeks Late: 6 months	tPA (100 mg) + IV Heparin Placebo + IV Heparin	7.2% 9.8% RRR 26% P=0.0011	10.4% 13.1% RRR 21% P=0.0026
LATE [14] 1993 Double-blind entry: 6–24 hours	5711 Early: 35 days Late: 12 months	tPA (100 mg) + IV Heparin + Aspirin Placebo + IV Heparin + Aspirin	8.9% 10.3% RRR 14% ns	14.0% 15.4% RRR 9.1% ns
EMERAS [15] 1993 Double-blind entry: 6–24 hours (protocol revision)	4534 Early: 35 days Late: 12 months	SK (1.5 MU) Placebo	13.2% 14.4% RRR 9% ns	18.9% 22.1% RRR 8% ns
EMIP [16] 1993 Double-blind entry: < 6 hours	5469 Early: pre-hospital Late: 30 days	APSAC (30 U) home/placebo hospital Placebo home/ APSAC hospital	1.3% 0.9% R.Excess R 44% ns	9.7% 11.1% RRR 13% P=0.08
GREAT [17,18] 1992, 94 Double-blind entry: < 4 hours	311 Early: in-hospital Late: 3 months	APSAC (30 U) home APSAC (30 U) hospital	6.7% 11.5% RRR 42%	10.4% 21.6% RRR 52% P=0.007

Table 3.2. Selected major studies of thrombolysis after myocardial infarction (MI). SK, streptokinase; MU, mega units; APSAC, anisoylated plasminogen-streptokinase activator complex; tPA, (recombinant) tissue plasminogen activator; RRR, relative risk reduction; U, units; IV, intravenous; ns, non-significant.

Streptokinase conferred the greatest advantage if administered within six hours of onset of pain [8,9], while some benefit could be obtained if given within 6–12 hours [8,15]. In the ISIS-II study, an additional benefit of reduced vascular deaths was found if aspirin was administered in conjunction with the streptokinase; the aspirin was also found to counter the slight excess of recurrent infarction from streptokinase administration alone [10]. The incidence of hypotension was slightly increased with streptokinase use. The risk of haemorrhagic stroke was also increased in the streptokinase group, but risk of ischaemic stroke was lessened; thus there was no overall change in risk of stroke.

Mortality may also be reduced by recombinant tissue plasminogen activator complex (tPA) therapy [12,13], although again an excess of reinfarction was found. The benefit of tPA is also conferred if patients are treated within 12 hours [14]. In the TIMI trial (phase I) [19] tPA was found to elicit reperfusion of infarct-related arteries twice as often as streptokinase.

In the AIMS study, anisoylated plasminogen-streptokinase activator complex (APSAC) reduced mortality in the year after infarction when given within six hours [11]. It is simple to use but is associated with an increase in recurrent infarction.

The EMIP study compared the administration of APSAC at home with that in hospital. Pre-hospital mortality tended to be higher in those given active therapy at home, but this was offset by greater benefit later on. In this study, the median time difference between pre- and in-hospital thrombolysis was only 30–60 minutes, too little to show a difference between strategies. In those patients where the delay was less than 90 minutes regardless of where thrombolysis was given, there was a 45% ($P < 0.05$) reduction in relative risk [16]. APSAC given by the general practitioner (GP) at home in the GREAT study saved an average time of two hours compared with hospital administration, and as such may reduce mortality by up to 50%; 15 patients had a cardiac arrest prior to hospital, most were resuscitated by their GPs and seven survived to discharge [17,18]. In a community-based (thus possibly less selective in patient recruitment) series of studies (MITI) [20–22], the overall risk of stroke with MI was 2.1%, and the incidence was unaffected by thrombolytic therapy. The rate of haemorrhagic, and therefore fatal, stroke was increased. Nevertheless, treatment within 70 minutes of symptom onset led to a reduction in mortality from 8.7 to 1.2% at 30 days ($P < 0.05$).

The Fibrinolytic Therapy Triallists [23] produced a meta-analysis including nine trials, with over 58 000 patients, which compared thrombolytic treatment with a control group. The following observations were made:
- Benefit was confirmed up to 12 hours after infarction. Evidence for benefit after the first 12 hours was smaller and statistically uncertain.
- Fibrinolytic therapy was associated with an excess in deaths in the first 24 hours, the risk increasing in elderly patients and those receiving treatment more than 12 hours after the onset of pain.
- No benefit was seen in those presenting with ST segment depression (although there were wide confidence intervals).

- Benefit was probably less with inferior infarction.
- More strokes occurred if treatment was delayed, age more than 75 years, blood pressure greater than 175 mmHg, previous MI or the initial ECG was normal or showed bundle branch block.

This overview allows subgroups at high risk of side effects and less benefit to be identified. Thus, for example, a patient older than 75 years presenting more than 12 hours after the onset of pain with an inferior infarct should not receive treatment without careful consideration.

Trials comparing thrombolytic agents

A summary of the studies is given in Table 3.3.

In the GISSI-II trial no difference in mortality was found using tPA and streptokinase. Favourable trends were observed for tPA in terms of reduced reinfarction and postinfarction angina but these were not significant. The tPA group had significantly less hypotension, fewer allergic reactions and fewer major bleeds. The trend to excess strokes with tPA was not significant [24].

In the ISIS-III trial no difference in mortality was found between the three treatment regimens [25]. APSAC was associated with a significantly greater risk of hypotension

Trials comparing thrombolytic agents				
Study	No. of patients Follow-up	Comparisons	Mortality	Stroke (fatal or disabling)
ISIS-II [10] 1988	17 187 5 weeks	SK Placebo	9.2% 12.0%	0.71% (0.5) 0.78% (0.6)
GISSI-II [24] 1990 Open label	12 490 In-hospital	SK tPA[†]	9.2% 9.6%	0.9% 1.1%
ISIS-III [25] 1992 Double-blind	41 299 in 3 groups 35 days and 6 months	SK APSAC tPA[†]	10.6% (14.0%) 10.5% (13.7%) 10.3% (14.1%)	1.04% (0.84%) 1.26% (1.08%) 1.39%* (1.13%)*
GUSTO [26] 1993 Open label	41 021 in 4 groups 30 days	SK + SC Heparin SK + IV Heparin Accelerated tPA + IV Heparin[††] SK + tPA + IV Heparin	7.2% 7.4% 6.3%** 7.0%	(Disabling only) 1.22% (0.5%) 1.40% (0.5%) 1.55% (0.6%) 1.64% (0.6%)

Table 3.3. Trials comparing thrombolytic agents (and data from ISIS-II for comparison). SK, streptokinase; tPA, tissue plasminogen activator complex; SC, subcutaneous; IV, intravenous; *$P < 0.05$, **$P < 0.001$. [†]See the ASSET trial for dosing regimen of tPA; [††]tPA given as 15 mg and 5000 units of heparin bolus, then 0.75 mg/kg tPA (maximum 50 mg) over 30 minutes, then 0.5 mg/kg tPA (maximum 35 mg) over 60 minutes and 1000 units heparin per hour (1200 units if patient > 80 kg).

and allergic reactions which were, however, generally mild. APSAC is given as a bolus, which may account for why these problems were observed most commonly in this group, compared with streptokinase which is given as an infusion that may be stopped early. There was a trend to excess stroke with APSAC but no difference in reinfarction. Allergic reactions and hypotension were less common with tPA and stroke was more common. There was no difference in major bleeding. In-hospital reinfarction was less common with tPA but this did not increase long-term survival.

The GUSTO trial showed a substantial reduction in mortality with tPA compared with other thrombolytic regimens [26]. The major differences between this trial and the others was the use of intravenous rather than subcutaneous heparin and the use of an accelerated dosing regimen for tPA. The use of tPA led to a non-significant increase in strokes and significant increases in haemorrhagic stroke. The accelerated tPA regimen was associated with fewer major bleeds, less heart failure and atrioventricular block, and fewer supraventricular and ventricular arrhythmias compared with the other intravenous heparin regimens. However, the incidence of reinfarction and major mechanical complications such as severe mitral regurgitation or ventricular septal defect was unaltered. Non-significant trends to even greater benefit with tPA compared with the streptokinase regimens were observed in younger patients and those with anterior infarcts, and significantly greater benefit was obtained in those treated within four hours.

Studies of secondary angioplasty

A summary of these trials is given in Table 3.4.

The ECSG study suggested a trend to excess mortality and morbidity with early angioplasty after tPA, even in those presenting within 2.5 hours of symptom onset [27]. The invasive strategy was associated with an increased risk of early recurrent ischaemia, and more hypotension and shock. Infarct size was not reduced and angiography performed about two weeks after infarction suggested no improvement in residual ventricular function with the invasive strategy. The SWIFT trial yielded a similar result, suggesting greater morbidity and longer hospital-stay among those randomized to angioplasty [30]. The TIMI-II trials also reported similar results and showed that routine delayed angiography with an intention to proceed to angioplasty was not superior to a conservative strategy [29]. The procedural mortality from percutaneous transluminal coronary angioplasty (PTCA) was 0.6% and 4.5% from procedure-related reinfarction. Patients receiving PTCA were less likely to need rehospitalization for cardiac reasons (38% v 30%, $P < 0.001$). The TOPS and TAMI trials [31,32], while hinting at possible subtle benefits of angioplasty, have produced no convincing argument for widespread use of angioplasty after MI.

Retrospective reports of series of patients with cardiogenic shock suggest that successful angioplasty is associated with a 70% chance of survival until discharge

Studies of secondary angioplasty			
Study	No. of patients Follow-up	Strategy	Mortality Early (Late)	Cumulative morbidity (%) CABG/MI/angina/PTCA (repeat PTCA)/CVA/CHF

Study	No. of patients Follow-up	Strategy	Mortality Early (Late)	Cumulative morbidity (%) CABG/MI/angina/PTCA (repeat PTCA)/CVA/CHF
ECSG 1988 [27]	367 14 days and 3 months	*Immediate angiography* Conservative	7% (8%) 3% (3%)	Cum. rate at 3 months 5/7/28/93(6)/0.5/? 6/10/30/15/0.5/?
TIMI-IIA 1990 [28]	586 6 weeks and (1 year)	*Immediate PTCA* Deferred PTCA *Conservative*	7.7% (8.2%) 5.7% (7.7%) 8.6% (10.2%)	Cum. rate at 12 months 19/10/18/76(1)/2/? 14/7/19/64(1)/2/? 18/10/21/24/2/?
TIMI-II 1992 [29]	3339 6 weeks and (1 year)	*Deferred PTCA* Conservative	5.2% (6.9%) 4.6% (7.4%)	Cum. rate at 12 months 18/9/24/61(1)/2/? 17/10/23/21/2/?
SWIFT 1991 [30]	800 12 months	*Early angiography* Conservative care	5.8 5.0%	17/15/19/42(0)/0/? 6/13/25/4/2/?
TOPS 1992 [31]	87 1 year	*Late PTCA* Conservative	0% (One patient died of cancer)	Cum. rate at 12 months 2/11/?/88(7)/0/5 2/0/?/9/0/7
TAMI 5 1987 [32]	575	*Immediate catheterization* Deferred catheterization	6% 4%	2+/3/25/18/2/14 ?/3/35/?/2/17

Table 3.4. CABG, coronary artery bypass graft; MI, myocardial infarction; PTCA, percutaneous transluminal coronary angioplasty; CVA, cerebrovascular accident; CHF, chronic heart failure. A question mark denotes data not available.

and 50% survival at one year versus 20–30% at both time-points among those with unsuccessful angioplasty [33,34]. Thrombolysis does not appear to influence outcome in this setting.

Studies of primary angioplasty

A summary is shown in Table 3.5.

Probably the first randomized trial of angioplasty was that by O'Neill *et al.*, who found encouraging "cosmetic" results in terms of angiography and ventricular function [35]. Nevertheless, deaths, post-infarction angina and need for surgery were similar in each group.

Later studies [36–38] established that angioplasty could be performed safely with few procedure-related deaths. Compared with thrombolysis (usually with tPA) the risk of stroke, reinfarction or major haemorrhage was lower with primary angioplasty. Angioplasty also led to a lower incidence of post-infarction angina, although delayed

Studies of primary angioplasty				
Study	No. of patients Follow-up	Comparison	Reinfarction Fatal and non-fatal	Mortality Early (late)
O'Neill 1986 [35] Prospective	56 7 months	*Immediate PTCA* Intracoronary streptokinase	$n=1$ $n=1$	$n=2$ $n=1$
Grines 1993 [36] Prospective	395 In-hospital (and 6 months)	*Immediate PTCA* IV tPA	2.6% (4.8%*) 6.5% (8.9%*)	2.6% (3.7%) 6.5% (7.9%)
Zijlstra 1993 [37] Prospective	142 In-hospital	*Immediate PTCA* IV streptokinase	$n=0$ $n=9$ $P=0.003$	$n=0$ $n=4$ ns
Gibbons 1993 [38] Prospective	108	*Immediate PTCA* IV tPA	$n=0$ $n=2$	$n=1$ $n=0$
Vacek 1992 [39] Retrospective observational	573 3 years (approx.)	*Primary angioplasty* Angioplasty after thrombolysis	5.7% 5.1%	17.9% 8.2% $P<0.001$

Table 3.5. PTCA, percutaneous transluminal coronary angioplasty; IV, intravenous; tPA, tissue plasminogen activator complex. *Non-fatal reinfarction only.

treatment may not be a worse option for managing this problem. Only one of the three studies suggested that PTCA led to greater preservation of ventricular function.

The use of thrombolysis followed by angioplasty has also been advocated [39], suggesting that angioplasty administered within 24 hours of thrombolysis may be especially useful. However, this was an uncontrolled study. Over 200 000 angioplasties were performed between 1987 and 1990 under the US Medicare system [40]. The overall in-hospital mortality for elective angioplasty was a little over 1%, but for angioplasty in the setting of acute infarction it rose to over 6.5%. Some of the high mortality could be attributed to attempted treatment of cardiogenic shock.

Studies involving surgical trials

The results of trials (Table 3.6) may be summarized as follows:
- In patients with a positive exercise test early after infarction, angiography and surgery for those with multivessel disease did not improve survival significantly [41].
- Coronary bypass surgery may be an option for patients with an evolving infarct and multivessel disease [44]. So long as the clinical picture (based on symptoms and ECG) was evolving, no critical time period for surgery was noted. No randomized study has been performed.
- The expected mortality from CABG at different times after infarction was

Surgical trials				
Trial	Timing	No. of patients Follow-up	Comparison	Mortality Early (late)
European CSBG 1992 [41] Randomized	Around 3 weeks post-MI	348 2 and 5 years	*Surgery* Medical therapy	7% 4% (12%) R.Excess R 75% at 2 years RRR 25% at 5 years
Norris 1981 and 1992 [42,43] Randomized	Around 5 months post-MI	200 1 and 10 years	*Surgery* Medical therapy	*6% (30%)* 7% (30%)
Phillips 1983 [44] Non-randomized	Evolving MI (including cardiogenic shock)	339 6.5 years	*Primary CABG* Streptokinase ± PTCA	*2.5%* 4.5%
Kennedy 1989 [45] Non-randomized	Within 30 days	793 Operative	*Day 1* Day 2–7 Day 8–30	*9.9%* *8.2%* *2.4%*
Bolooki 1989 [46] Non-randomized	Cardiogenic shock	200+ Up to 5 years	*Acute MI* Failed PTCA *Failed PTCA + streptokinase* Due to MR *Due to VSD* Ruptured free wall *Arrhythmia-induced*	36% (90%)* 17% 29% 46% (40%)* 55% (84%)* 45% 50% (66%)*
Barner 1989 [47] Non-randomized	No cardiogenic shock	1897 Up to 1 year	*Failed PTCA* Poststreptokinase Primary	*3.6% (38% MI)** 2.8% 4.9%

Table 3.6. MI, myocardial infarction; R.Excess R, relative excess risk; RRR, relative risk reduction; CABG, coronary artery bypass graft; PTCA, percutaneous transluminal coronary angioplasty; MR, mitral regurgitation; VSD, ventricular septal defect. *Percentage surviving for at least one year among those that survive surgery; **rate of peri-operative MI.

studied [45]. Female sex, age greater than 60 years, Q-wave infarction, heart failure, need for emergency surgery and previous CABG all increased risk significantly.

- About one-half of patients with cardiogenic shock survive after emergency revascularization regardless of whether it is caused by ventricular septal defect, mitral regurgitation or primary myocardial dysfunction [46]. The long-term survival of those surviving the first month is good (80–90%), apart from those with shock arising from mitral regurgitation (40%).
- Operation within 12 hours of thrombolysis is associated with increased bleeding that may require transfusion or reoperation.

The effects of anti-arrhythmic agents after myocardial infarction

These are summarized in Table 3.7.

Effects of anti-arrhythmic agents after MI				
Study	No. of patients Follow-up	Comparisons	VF or sudden death	Mortality
IMPACT 1984 [48]	630 12 months	*Mexilitene* Placebo	$n=7$ $n=4$	7.6% 4.8% R.Excess R 58% ns
N-NLIT 1992 [49]	204 Pre-hospital	*LIgnocaine* Placebo	$n=5$ $n=3$	$n=1$ $n=1$
Tocainide 1983 [50]	791 48 hours	*Tocainide* Placebo	Primary VF $n=11$ $n=6$	$n=9$ $n=8$
CAST-I 1989, 1991 [51,52]	1 455 10 months	*Encainide/ Flecainide* Placebo	4.5% 1.2% R.Excess R 375% P=0.0006	7.7% 3.0% R.Excess R 257% P<0.0003
CAST-II 1992 [53]	1 374 18 months	*Moricizine* Placebo	9.7% 5.7% R.Excess R 70% ns	15.1% 12.6% R.Excess R 20% ns
Ceremuzynski 1992 [54] Double-blind	613 12 months	*Amiodarone* Placebo	Data unavailable	6.9% 10.7% RRR 36% ns
BASIS 1990, 1993 [55,56] Open label	212 72 months	*Amiodarone for first 12 months only* Placebo for first 12 months	4.1% (1.1% pa)* 8.8% (1.6% pa)* RRR 53% P<0.05	5.1% (2.6% pa)* 11.4% (4.1% pa)* RRR 55% P<0.05
Navarro-Lopez 1993 [57] Open label	368 2.8 years	*Amiodarone* Metoprolol Control	$n=3$ $n=9$ $n=5$	$n=4$ (3.5%) $n=17$ (15.4%) $n=9$ (7.7%)

Table 3.7. VF, ventricular fibrillation; R.Excess R, relative excess risk; RRR, relative risk reduction. *Mortality rates per annum excluding the first year after myocardial infarction (MI).

In the CAST-I study patients with impaired ventricular function could be entered between six days and two years after infarction (78% were entered within 90 days) if they had more than six ectopics per hour on Holter monitoring [51,52]. This trial revolutionized our view of anti-arrhythmic drugs, emphasizing the need to assess meaningful endpoints such as survival rather than surrogates such as arrhythmia suppression. It is worth remembering that patients were initially challenged with flecainide or encainide and could not enter the study if a pro-arrhythmic effect was observed. Patients exhibiting a pro-arrhythmic response to a class I agent had a worse prognosis than those who did not, perhaps because pro-arrhythmia is itself a marker of poor ventricular function and a worse prognosis. It is worth noting that about one-third of the CAST population were receiving diuretics, presumably mostly for heart failure, and that these patients had a mortality about four times that of the rest of the population. In other words, most of the excess deaths in the CAST patients were among those with heart failure.

The results of other studies and meta-analysis suggest that class I agents in general, including mexiletine, lignocaine, tocainide and moricizine, do not prevent ventricular fibrillation and may have a deleterious effect on survival post-MI.

In contrast, meta-analysis suggests that amiodarone may reduce mortality after MI. The BASIS study selected patients who had complex non-sustained arrhythmias after MI, and found that amiodarone appeared better in terms of improving survival than did either no anti-arrhythmic treatment or treatment tailored by Holter monitoring in individual patients. The investigators stopped therapy after 12 months and found no excess mortality in those withdrawn from amiodarone [55,56]. Patients with poor ventricular function appeared to have less benefit with amiodarone. Amiodarone is generally well tolerated but induced a bradycardia (possibly helpful) or thyrotoxicosis in 4% of cases [54]. Disappointingly, unlike the beta blockers, it does not appear to reduce reinfarction.

Meta-analysis suggests that beta blockers may be the most successful agents for reducing sudden cardiac death [58–60].

The early use of beta blockers post-myocardial infarction

A summary of studies is given in Table 3.8.

The first study to show conclusively that very early administration of a beta blocker could reduce mortality after MI was by Hjalmarson et al. [61]. Metoprolol also appeared to reduce infarct size.

Propranolol given by the family doctor, prior to hospital, to patients with suspected MI reduced the frequency of ventricular fibrillation prior to or in hospital, although total mortality was unaffected [62]. Progression from threatened to completed infarction was also unaffected. Very early administration of a beta blocker was found to reduce the risk of sudden death, but not overall mortality,

Early use of beta blockers post-MI with and without long-term treatment				
Study	No. of patients Follow-up	Comparisons	Sudden (arrhythmic) death	Total mortality
Hjalmarson 1981 [61] Double-blind	1395 3 months	IV + oral metoprolol Placebo	0.9% 2.4% RRR 62% P<0.01	5.7% 8.9% RRR 36% P<0.03
PREMIS 1984 [62] Open label	735 Pre- and in-hospital	IV + oral propanolol No beta blocker	n=2 n=14 P=0.006	n=15 n=14
Salathia 1985 [63] Double-blind	800 12 months	IV + oral metoprolol Placebo	1.9% 4.7% RRR 60% P=0.05	11.9% 13.6% RRR 12% ns
MIAMI 1985 [64] Double-blind	5778 15 days	IV + oral metoprolol Placebo	No significant effect on VT or VF	4.3% 4.9% RRR 12% ns
ISIS-I 1981 [65] Open label	16027 7 days and 1 year	IV + oral atenolol No beta blocker	2.4% 2.5% RRR 4% ns	3.9% (10.7%) 4.6% (12.0%) RRR 15% (11%) P<0.04 (P<0.01)
TIMI-IIB 1991 [66] Open label	1434 6 days and 1 year	IV + oral metoprolol No therapy until day 6, oral metoprolol thereafter	n=5 n=9	2.4% (4.8%) 2.4% (5.0%) ns

Table 3.8. Major studies with early use of beta blockers post-myocardial infarction (MI) with and without long-term treatment. IV, intravenous; RRR, relative risk reduction; VT, ventricular tachycardia; VF, ventricular fibrillation. IV dose of metoprolol 15 mg and of atenolol 5–10 mg.

in another study [63]. Primary ventricular fibrillation was rare and was not significantly reduced by the beta blocker.

An overall benefit for the early use of metoprolol after MI was not shown in the MIAMI trial [64]. Among high-risk patients, metoprolol appeared to be of some benefit (29% relative risk reduction [RRR]; P<0.04). Early metoprolol use appeared to reduce infarct size and prevent 2–3% of threatened infarcts from evolving.

The benefit from atenolol was confined largely to the first 24 hours in ISIS-I [65]. An analysis of the causes of death suggested that atenolol could reduce the risk of cardiac rupture, although this was not corroborated by the MIAMI trial. Cardiac arrest and reinfarction were not significantly reduced. There was no evidence that atenolol could abort a threatened infarct.

The TIMI-IIB study failed to show a marked advantage of very early (compared with later) introduction of a beta blocker in patients who had received tPA. However, the major cause of death in patients considered at low risk in the first six days was arrhythmia, and this was completely abolished by early beta blockade. Cardiac rupture and heart failure were not altered by early beta blocker use. Patients receiving tPA within two hours of chest pain seemed to benefit more from early beta blockade [66].

Meta-analysis suggests about a 15% reduction in overall mortality in the first week, mostly in the first 24 hours (about four lives saved for every 1000 treated for one day). There was about an 18% reduction in reinfarction and a 15% reduction in ventricular fibrillation [65,67].

Late initiation and long-term beta blocker use post-myocardial infarction

A summary of these trials is given in Table 3.9.

The Norwegian timolol trial was the first to show convincingly the benefits of long-term beta blockade on mortality, mainly due to reductions in reinfarction and sudden death [68]. The benefits were independent of age, and were shown to be similar in high- and low-risk groups, although the absolute benefits were greatest in those at highest risk. Beta blockade confers a reduced mortality even after six years [69], indicating either that beta blockade irrevocably alters prognosis after MI or that there is continuing benefit from long-term beta blockade.

The long-term use of propranolol has also been shown to reduce overall mortality, largely by a reduction in sudden death [71,72]. There was also a downward trend in non-fatal reinfarction but a slightly increased risk of developing heart failure, but only in the first two weeks of administration. Patients with and without heart failure had a similar mortality benefit from propranolol; since the group with heart failure had a higher mortality, the absolute benefits in this group were greater.

When beta blockers with intrinsic sympathomimetic activity are used, they show no benefit and possible evidence of harm [70,74] with the exception of the APSI study [77]. The LIT trial used a selective beta blocker but results were generally less impressive than the trials with non-selective beta blockers [75]. Sotalol does not seem to confer unusual benefit on outcomes such as arrhythmias or sudden death. Although the reduction in reinfarction was striking in the trial by Julian (Sotalol Trial), numbers were quite small [73].

In the longest randomized follow-up of any of the beta blocker trials [76], the overall benefits of treatment appeared to increase with time. However, patients with small infarcts had a good prognosis that was not improved by treatment, while older

Later initiation and long-term use of beta blockers post-MI				
Study	No. of patients Follow-up	Comparisons	Reinfarction (fatal and non-fatal)	Total mortality (sudden death)
Norwegian Multicentre 1981 [68,69] Double-blind	1884 17 months (average)	Timolol (10 mg bd) Placebo	14.4% 20.1% RRR 28.4%	10.6% (5.0%) 17.5% (10.1%) RRR 39% P=0.0005
Australian/ Swedish 1983 [70] Double-blind	529 2 years	Pindolol (15 mg/day) Placebo	14.1% 15.4% RRR 8% ns	17.1% (10.6%) 17.7% (11.7%) RRR 5% ns
BHAT 1983 [71,72] Double-blind	3837 2 years	Propranolol (60–80 mg tid) Placebo	Non-fatal only 4.4% 5.3% RRR 16% ns	7.2% (3.3%) 9.8% (4.6%) RRR 26% P<0.005
Julian 1982 [73] Double-blind	1456 12 months	Sotalol (320 mg/day) Placebo	3.3% 5.7% RRR 41% P<0.05	7.3% (4.3%) 8.9% (3.&%)* RRR 18% ns
EIS group 1984 [74] Double-blind Open label	1741 12 months	Oxprenolol (160 mg bd) Placebo	6.2% 5.1% R.Excess R 22% ns	6.6% (2.9%) 5.1% (2.7%) R.Excess R 29% ns
LIT 1987 [75] Double-blind	2395 18 months	Metoprolol (100 mg bd) Placebo	ND	7.2% 7.8% RRR 8% ns
Olsson 1985 [76]	301 36 months	Metoprolol (100 mg bd) Placebo	Non-fatal only 11.7% 21.1% RRR 45% P<0.05	16.2% (5.8%) 21.1% (14.3%) RRR 23% (59%) ns (P<0.05)
APSI 1990 [77] Double-blind	607 10 months	Acebutolol (200 mg bd) Placebo	3.0% 3.6% RRR 17% ND	5.7% 11.0% RRR 48% P<0.01

Table 3.9. Major studies with later initiation (2–36 days) and long-term use of beta blockers post-myocardial infarction (MI). RRR, relative risk reduction; R.Excess R, relative excess risk; ND, no data. *Sudden death, death within one hour of symptoms or timing of death in relation to symptoms unknown.

patients and those with large infarcts obtained most benefit. Interestingly, metoprolol seemed more effective in reducing not only mortality but also reinfarction among those with a large MI.

On meta-analysis where beta blockade was initiated late, the placebo versus active treatment mortality is 10.1% versus 8.0% (RRR 21%; $P < 0.0001$). However, this ranges from a RRR of 39% in the timolol trials to a relative excess risk (R.Excess R) of 29% with oxprenolol in the EIS trial [68,69,74].

Although meta-analysis has not been able to confirm that these differences are statistically meaningful, it seems wise to avoid beta blockers with high intrinsic sympathomimetic activity (ISA). There is no evidence of additional mortality benefits from using sotalol or a selective beta blocker, though ancillary properties may be useful or minimize side effects. However, post-infarction hypokalaemia seems less frequent with non-selective beta blockers, an effect on the beta-2-receptor, and this may give non-selective beta blockers an advantage [78].

Placebo-controlled trials of calcium antagonists post-myocardial infarction

The major placebo-controlled trials of calcium antagonists post-MI are shown in Table 3.10.

The first mega-trial with a calcium antagonist (TRENT) failed to show a benefit in mortality at 28 days [80]. The SPRINT-I study also failed to show a difference between placebo and nifedipine [81]. The SPRINT-II study was conducted in high-risk patients only, with a higher dose of nifedipine in view of the neutral outcome in SPRINT I. The study was stopped prematurely owing to an increase in overall mortality during the first week in those randomized to nifedipine. However, the risk of sudden death tended to be less frequent in the nifedipine-treated group [82].

A trial of diltiazem on patients with non-Q-wave MI [83] suggested a marked reduction in the risk of reinfarction, but a trend to increased mortality. Of the patients studied, 61% received concomitant beta blockers. Diltiazem also reduced the frequency of refractory post-infarction angina by 50% ($P < 0.05$). In the MDPIT study diltiazem, started 3–15 days after MI, exerted no overall benefit [84]. However, if patients with radiological evidence of heart failure were excluded there was a 23% reduction in cardiac events.

When verapamil was compared with placebo in the DAVIT-I study, it failed to show an overall effect. Within the first week verapamil appeared harmful; however, use of verapamil thereafter was associated with significant reductions in mortality and reinfarction [85]. In the DAVIT-II study a downward trend in mortality and a statistically significant reduction in reinfarction were found when verapamil was started a mean of nine days after infarction [86]. Verapamil did not change mortality in patients with heart failure but reduced overall mortality in those without heart failure ($P < 0.02$) in a prespecified subgroup analysis [87].

Meta-analysis of the calcium antagonist trials [87] suggests potential harm with nifedipine, a fairly neutral effect on mortality for diltiazem and a trend to benefit with

Placebo-controlled trials of calcium antagonists post-MI				
Study	No. of patients Follow-up	Comparisons	Reinfarction	Mortality (sudden death)
Belfast 1988 [79] Double-blind	434 2 days	Nifedipine (60 mg/day) Placebo	ND	6.6% 5.8% R.Excess R 14% ns
TRENT 1986 [80] Double-blind	4491 28 days	Nifedipine (40 mg/day) Placebo	2.2% 1.5% R.Excess R 47% ns	6.7% 6.3% R.Excess R 7% ns
SPRINT-I 1988 [81] Double-blind	2276 10 months	Nifedipine (30 mg/day) Placebo	6.4% 6.5% RRR 2% ns	5.8% (2.0%) 5.7% (2.4%) R.Excess R 2% (RRR 17%) ns
SPRINT-II 1993 [82] Double-blind	1373 6 months	Nifedipine (60 mg/day) Placebo	Non-fatal only 5.1% 4.2% R.Excess R 21% ns	18.7% (2.3%) 15.6% (4.9%) R.Excess R 20% (RRR 53%) ns
Diltiazem Reinfarction Study 1986 [83] Double-blind	576 14 days	Diltiazem (360 mg/day) Placebo	5.2% 9.3% RRR 51% P<0.03	3.8% 3.1% R.Excess R 23% ns
MDPIT 1988 [84] Double-blind	2466 25 months	Diltiazem (120–240 mg/day) Placebo	Non-fatal only 8.0% 9.4% RRR 15% ns	13.5% 13.5% RRR 0% ns
DAVIT-I 1984 [85] Double-blind	1436 (with confirmed MI) 12 months	IV + oral verapamil Placebo	7.8% 9.2% RRR 15% ns	15.2% (4.9%) 16.4% (6.0%) RRR 7% ns
DAVIT-II 1991 [86,87] Double-blind	1775 16 months (average)	Oral verapamil (360 mg/day) Placebo	11.0% 13.2% RRR 17% P<0.04	11.1% 13.8% RRR 20% ns

Table 3.10. MI, myocardial infarction; ND, no data; R.Excess R, relative risk reduction; RRR, relative risk reduction.

verapamil. There is doubt about the benefit of diltiazem for non-Q-wave infarction. Verapamil may be a useful substitute for a beta blocker in patients with asthma or other contraindications to a beta blocker but must be avoided in patients with heart failure.

The short-term early-entry aspirin trials

These are summarized in Table 3.11.

Short-term early-entry aspirin trials					
Study	No. of patients Follow-up	Comparisons	Reinfarction	Stroke	Total mortality
ISIS-II [10]	17 187	Aspirin (162.5 mg/day)	1.8%	0.5%	9.5%
Double-blind	35 days	Placebo	3.3% RRR 46% P<0.0001	0.9% RRR 44% P<0.01	12.0% RRR 21% P=0.00001
RISK [88]	796	Aspirin (75 mg) Placebo	Non-fatal MI 2.3% (5.0%) 5.5% (14.6%) RRR 58% (66%) ns (P<0.001)	? None	n=1 (1.5%) n=1 (2.5%) RRR 0% (40%) ns (ns)
Double-blind	5 days and (3 months)				

Table 3.11. Figures in parentheses indicate late events. RRR, relative risk reduction; MI, myocardial infarction.

In the ISIS-II study it was established conclusively that aspirin should be given immediately after MI and continued for at least three to four weeks thereafter [10]. Aspirin was effective in most subgroups. However, in patients who had suffered more than one infarction, aspirin was ineffective. In patients with unstable angina or non-Q-wave infarction in the RISK study, aspirin was highly beneficial in preventing recurrent infarction [88].

Long-term aspirin trials

A summary of trials is given in Table 3.12.

The long-term aspirin studies have been disappointing. The trends to reduction even in non-fatal infarction have generally not been significant and not accompanied by a reduction in mortality. Indeed, the disparity between reinfarction and mortality (with a trend to increased sudden death on aspirin) may reflect the analgesic properties of aspirin and an increase in the proportion of silent MI. The trend to an excess mortality in patients with heart failure treated with aspirin indicates the need to establish the safety of this treatment in this subgroup [97,98].

Most of the studies used aspirin 1000 mg per day or more. There is no substantial post-

Long-term aspirin trials					
Study	No. of patients Follow-up	Comparisons	Reinfarction	Stroke	Total mortality
Cardiff-I 1974 [89] Double-blind	1239 12 months	Aspirin (300 mg/day) Placebo	ND	ND	8.3% 10.9% RRR 24% ns
Cardiff-II 1979 [90] Double-blind	1682 12 months	Aspirin (300 mg tid) Placebo	10.9% 7.1% RRR 34% ns	ND	12.3% 14.8% RRR 17% ns
CDP-A 1988 [91] Double-blind	1259 (men) 22 months	Aspirin (324 mg tid) Placebo	8.0% 10.2% RRR 21% ns	0.9% 1.2% RRR 25% ns	5.8% 8.3% RRR 30% ns
AMIS 1980 [92,93] Double-blind	4524 38 months	Aspirin (500 mg tid) Placebo	9.5% 11.6% RRR 18% ns	1.4% 2.2% RRR 36% ns 1.1%	10.8% 9.7% R.Excess R 11% ns
PARIS-I 1980 [94,95] Double-blind	2026 41 months	Aspirin (324 mg tid) Placebo	6.9% 9.9% RRR 30% $P<0.05$	2.0% RRR 45% ns 1.3%	10.5% 12.8% RRR 18% ns
PARIS-II 1987 [96] Double-blind	3128 23 months	Dipyridamole + Aspirin (330 mg tid) Placebo	9.0% 11.8% RRR 24% ns	2.3% RRR 43% ns	7.1% 7.3% RRR 3% ns

Table 3.12. ND, no data; tid, three times per day; *ns,* non-significant; RRR, relative risk reduction.

MI study with aspirin 75 mg per day. There were 139 vascular deaths in the four substantial studies in other vascular conditions conducted with aspirin 75 mg per day but only 150 in the control groups (non-significant) [97,98]. Vascular deaths in the primary prevention studies were 238 on aspirin versus 250 in the control group (non-significant) [97,98].

The US Physicians study suggested a reduction in first infarction with the use of aspirin, but as there was no difference in vascular deaths (91 aspirin versus 92 control) and an excess of sudden death in the aspirin group, this may reflect an increase in the proportion of unrecognized MI in the aspirin group.

Studies comparing aspirin and coumarin

A summary of trials is given in Table 3.13.

Studies comparing aspirin and coumarin					
Study	No. of patients Follow-up	Comparisons	Non-fatal reinfarction	Stroke	Total mortality
GAMIS 1980 [99] Aspirin double-blind, Coumarin open label	946 24 months	*Coumarin* Aspirin (1500 mg) Placebo	*1.9%* 3.5% 4.9% *ns*	*None* None None	*12.2%* 8.5% 10.4% *ns*
EPSIM 1982 [100] Open label	1303 29 months	*Coumarin* Aspirin (500 mg tid)	*3.1%* 4.9% *ns*	*0.8%* 0.5% *ns*	*10.0%* 11.0% *ns*

Table 3.13. *ns*, non-significant.

The GAMIS trial failed to show significant differences in outcome with the use of aspirin or phenprocoumon [99]. The EPSIM trial showed that patients were less likely to withdraw from anticoagulation with full dose warfarin than high-dose aspirin [100]. Trends in favour of the anticoagulant were not significant.

Short-term coumarin trials

A summary is given in Table 3.14.

Short-term coumarin trials					
Study	No. of patients Follow-up	Comparisons	Reinfarction	Stroke	Total mortality
MRC 1969 [101] Open label	1427 28 days	*Heparin then full-dose phenindione* Low-dose phenindione only	*9.7%* 13.0% RRR 25% *ns*	*1.1%* 2.5% RRR 25% $P<0.01$	*16.2%* 18.0% RRR 10% *ns*
Veterans 1973 [102] Open label	999 28 days	*Heparin then warfarin* Placebo then placebo	*3.4%* 4.8% RRR 29% *ns*	*0.8%* 3.2% RRR 75% $P<0.001$	*9.6%* 11.2% RRR 14% *ns*

Table 3.14. RRR, relative risk reduction; *ns*, non-significant.

The MRC trial showed a trend to less reinfarction and death, and a significant reduction in stroke in patients treated with the more aggressive anticoagulant regimen [101]. Thirty-six patients had a haemorrhagic episode, four times higher than the rate in the low-dose group. The Veterans Trial failed to show a benefit on short-term mortality after MI [102]. Favourable trends for less reinfarction and heart failure were not significant. The risk of stroke, pulmonary embolism and other vascular occlusion was lower in the warfarin group. Major bleeding was no more common in the anticoagulated group.

Long-term coumarin trials

A summary of long-term coumarin trials is given in Table 3.15.

The MRC long-term study was designed with the premise that intensive anti-coagulation would reduce mortality by 75%. It failed to do so but did reduce mortality by 33%, although this was not statistically significant [103]. There were 16 potentially serious haemorrhagic episodes over more than 5000 patient months in

Long-term coumarin trials					
Study	No. of patients Follow-up	Comparisons	Reinfarction	Stroke	Total mortality
MRC 1964 [103] Open label	383 5 years	High-dose phenindione Low-dose phenindione	43.1% 17.4% RRR 60%	Data not available	21.3% 14.9% RRR 30%
Veterans 1969 [104] Open label	731 2 years and 5 years	Warfarin No warfarin	(15.6%) (20.9%) RRR (25%) ns	Data not given	11.4% (27.0%) 17.1% (28.9%) RRR 33% (7%) P<0.01 (ns)
Sixty Plus Reinfarction Study 1982 [105] Double-blind	878 24 months	Coumarin Placebo	6.6% 14.6% RRR 45% P=0.0005	2.7% 4.6% RRR 41% ns	11.6% 15.7% RRR 26% P=0.07
WARIS 1990 [106] Double-blind	1214 37 months	Warfarin Placebo	13.5% 20.4% RRR 34% P=0.0007	3.3% 7.2% RRR 55% P=0.0015	15.5% 20.3% RRR 24% P=0.027
ASPECT 1994 [107] Double-blind	3404 37 months	Coumarin Placebo	6.7% 14.2% RRR 47% P<0.001	2.2% 3.6% RRR 39% P<0.01	10% 11.1% RRR 10% ns

Table 3.15. RRR, relative risk reduction; *ns*, non-significant.

the high-dose group compared with none in the low dose group. The Veterans long-term study showed a favourable effect of warfarin on survival for the first four years [104]. The benefit of warfarin appeared to wane with time. There were four deaths due to bleeding. Warfarin reduced reinfarction (*see* opposite) and heart failure (7.0% v 13.1%; $P<0.01$). Patients not treated with anticoagulants had a higher disability score. The Sixty Plus reinfarction study withdrew patients over the age of 60 years who had been receiving anticoagulants for at least six months after MI (the mean time from infarction to withdrawal was almost six years) [105]. This was the first study to show a conclusive effect of anticoagulants on reinfarction although not on mortality on an intention-to-treat basis. However, among those who took the anti-coagulant as prescribed there was a 43% reduction in all cause mortality ($P<0.02$). In the WARIS study warfarin was started about one month after infarction [106]. This is the only study that has shown a clear-cut reduction in mortality with the use of warfarin or, indeed, any antithrombotic agent used long-term post-MI. A powerful effect of warfarin on reinfarction and stroke was also demonstrated. Only eight patients had a major extracranial bleed. The target International Normalized Ratio (INR) was 2.8–4.8. The ASPECT study showed that anticoagulation could reduce major morbidity after MI though there was no clear-cut reduction in mortality [107]. The target INR was 2.8–4.8, and 1.5% of patients receiving active treatment had a major haemorrhage (versus 0.2% of control).

Heparin trials

A summary is given in Table 3.16.

Overall the evidence of a reduction in mortality with the use of high-dose subcutaneous heparin is dubious; any effect is small and associated with an excess risk of haemorrhagic stroke. The use of intravenous heparin appears even more hazardous [25]. The need for intravenous heparin with accelerated tPA, as suggested in the GUSTO trial, remains to be substantiated. Serneri *et al.* administered low-dose subcutaneous (SC) heparin long term to post-MI patients; he suggested that chronic heparin therapy reduced reinfarction and possibly mortality [109, 110].

Magnesium trials

A summary is given in Table 3.17.

The reasons for the difference in outcome between the LIMIT-II and ISIS-IV studies with respect to the effects of magnesium are disputed. The magnesium was given earlier in LIMIT-II, at a mean of three hours after the onset of pain, and before spont-aneous or therapeutic thrombolysis was likely. Thus, magnesium may have

Heparin trials					
Study	No. of patients Follow-up	Comparison	Reinfarction	Stroke	Total mortality Early (late)
ISIS-III 1992 [25] Open label	41 299 in 3 groups 35 days and 6 months	SC Heparin* Control	3.2% 3.5% RRR 9% ns	1.3% 1.2% R.Excess R 8% ns	10.3% (13.9%) 10.6% (14%) RRR 3% ns
GISSI-II 1992 [24] Open label	12 490 In-hospital and 6 months	SC Heparin Control	1.9% 2.3% RRR 16% ns	1.0% 1.0%	9.3% 9.4% RRR 11% ns
GUSTO 1993 [26] Open label	20 251 30 days	SK + IV Heparin SK + SC Heparin	4.0% 3.4% R.Excess R 18% ns	0.8% 0.7% R.Excess R 14% ns	7.4% 7.2% R.Excess R 3% ns
RISK 1990 [85] Double-blind	796 5 days and (3 months)	IV Bolus Heparin (5000 units qid) in hospital ± Aspirin Placebo ± Aspirin	No clear benefit	? None	Deaths and MI 3.4% (11.0%) 4.9% (12.6%) RRR 31% (12%) ns
SCATI 1989 [108] Open label	711 In-hospital	IV Heparin (2000 units) + 12 500 units bd Control	Non-fatal 5.5% 6.8% RRR 19% ns	n = 0 n = 2	5.8% 9.9% RRR 41% P < 0.03
Serneri 1987, 1993 [109,110] Open label	728 9 months (average)	SC Heparin (12 500 units day) Control	1.4% 3.6% RRR 61% P = 0.05	n = 0 n = 2	4.1% 6.3% RRR 35% ns

Table 3.16. SC, subcutaneous; RRR, relative risk reduction; R.Excess R, relative excess risk ; MI, myocardial infarction; *ns*, non-significant. *Heparin (12 500 units bd) given with aspirin and antithrombolytic.

reduced reperfusion injury, improving ventricular function and reducing heart failure deaths [111,112]. In contrast, magnesium was given at a mean of eight hours after the onset of symptoms, and after streptokinase had been given in ISIS-IV. Magnesium caused an excess of hypotension in ISIS-IV and there was a possible deleterious interaction with captopril (ISIS-IV: oral communication from the European Society of Cardiology Meeting on Heart Failure, Glasgow, 1994). Thus, magnesium may have caused infarct extension in some patients. The LIMIT-II investigators suggest that delays in the administration of magnesium may have led to the poor result. Although meta-analysis of small studies in the pre-thrombolytic era (most of which were positive) supports a reduction in mortality, this was generally considered

Magnesium trials					
Study	No. of patients Follow-up	Comparisons	Arrhythmia	Heart failure	Mortality
LIMIT-II 1992 [111,112]	2316	Mg (8 mmol/5 min) then 65 mmol over 24 hours)	Excess sinus Bradycardia No reduction in VF	11.2%	7.8% (22.8%)
Double-blind	28 days and (2.7 years)	Placebo		14.9% RRR 25% P=0.009	10.3% (26.5%) RRR 24% (16%) P=0.04 (P=0.03)
ISIS-IV 1995 [113]	~58 000	Mg (8 mmol/ 15 min, then 72 mmol over 24 hours)	3.5%	17.9%	7.8% (10.3%)
Open label	35 days and (6 months)	Control	3.8% RRR 8% ns	16.7% R.Excess R 7% ns	7.3% (10.2%) R.Excess R 6% (1%) ns
Galloe 1993 [114] Double-blind	468 1 year	Oral mg 15 mmol/day Placebo	6.8% 5.6% R.Excess R 21% ns	15.7% 11.6% R.Excess R 35% ns	13.1% 8.4% R.Excess R 56% ns

Table 3.17. Mg, magnesium; VF, ventricular fibrillation; RRR, relative risk reduction; *ns*, non-significant; R.Excess R, relative excess risk.

to be due to a reduction in arrhythmias [113]. The finding that heart failure deaths, but not arrhythmias, were reduced in LIMIT-II indicates a general lack of consensus in the result of magnesium trials.

The study by Galloe *et al.* [114] suggests that long-term oral magnesium supplements after MI may actually be harmful ($P=0.02$ for the combined cardiovascular morbidity and mortality). The oral and intravenous studies are not comparable for several reasons, including the fact that oral magnesium supplements may not increase plasma magnesium concentration.

Trials using ACE inhibitors

A summary of trials using ACE inhibitors is given in Table 3.18.

The CONSENSUS-II study achieved rapid ACE inhibition by use of intravenous enalapril in patients with definite MI and continued oral enalapril for six months; patients with systolic pressure less than 105 mmHg were excluded [115]. The study was abandoned early as it was felt that the outcome would be neutral using the planned study size and duration. Even so, there was evidence that enalapril reduced the number of patients progressing to heart failure; longer-term follow-up might

Trials of ACE inhibitors					
Study	No. of patients Follow-up	Comparison	Reinfarction	Heart failure	Mortality
CONSENSUS -II 1992 [115]	6090	IV Enalapril + Oral (10 mg bd)	8.9%	26.6%	10.2%
Double-blind	6 months	Placebo	8.8% R.Excess R 1% ns	29.8% RRR 11% P=0.006	9.4% R.Excess R 9% ns
SAVE 1992 [116] Double-blind	2231 42 months (average)	Captopril (50 mg tid) Placebo	9.7% 11.6% RRR 16% ns	10.6% 16.0% RRR 37% P<0.001	20.4% 24.6% RRR 19% P=0.014
AIRE 1993 [117] Double-blind	2006 15 months (average)	Ramipril (5 mg bd) Placebo	8.1% 9.0% RRR 11% ns	14.2% 18.1% RRR 22% P=0.008˙	16.9% 22.6% RRR 27% P<0.002
PRACTICAL 1994 [118] Double-blind	225 3 and (12 months)	Enalapril 5 mg tid Captopril 25 mg tid Placebo	ND	Not given	n=1˙˙ (2)[†] n=9˙˙ (10)[†] n=7˙˙ (12)[†] P<0.04˙˙ (P<0.03)[†]
SMILE 1995 [119] Double-blind	1556 42 days	Zofenopril 30 mg bd Placebo	n=11 n=12 RRR 7% ns	8.9% 13.6% RRR 35% P<0.01	6.5% 8.3% RRR 22% ns
TRACE 1995 [120] Double-blind	1749 2 or more years	Trandolapril 4 mg Placebo	Not yet reported	Not yet reported	34.7% 42.3% RRR 22%[††] P<0.01
ISIS-IV 1994 [121] Double-blind	54 824 35 days and (6 months)	Captopril 50 mg bd Placebo	4.1% 3.9%	17.1% 17.4%	6.9% (9.9%) 7.3% (10.6%)[††] RR 6% (7%) P=0.04
GISSI-III 1994 [122] Open label	19 394 42 days	Lisinopril (10 mg od) control	3.2% 3.1% R. Excess R 3% ns	3.9% 3.7% R.Excess R 5% ns	6.3% 7.1% RRR 11% P=0.03

Table. 3.18. ACE, angiotensin-converting enzyme; IV, intravenous; bd, twice daily; R.Excess R, relative excess risk; RRR, relative risk reduction; tid, three times daily; ns, non-significant; ND, no data. ˙A major contributor to combined endpoint; ˙˙early mortality; [†]late mortality; [††]as at June 1994.

have seen this translated into a mortality benefit. The trialists have made detailed arguments that the initial hypotension was a marker of risk but not the cause of increased mortality (possibly by increasing infarct size and early deaths); these arguments are unconvincing.

Patients were entered into the SAVE study a mean of 11 days after infarction if the LVEF was less than 40% by RNVG. Patients who had evidence of ischaemia at rest or on an exercise test had to have angiography prior to entry; and if PTCA or CABG was deemed necessary, this had also to be performed before entry [116]. It is of note that the mortality in US and Canadian centres was similar, though the coronary intervention rate was very much higher in the USA. This was the first study to show a conclusive reduction in mortality with the use of an ACE inhibitor after MI. Mortality was reduced by effects both on progressive heart failure and on sudden death. Reinfarction, rather than progressive dilatation, was possibly the most important cause of worsening heart failure, although whether the reduction in non-fatal reinfarction with captopril achieved statistical significance is disputed.

The outcomes of SAVE and CONSENSUS-II are compatible; no benefit was observed in SAVE until the second year of follow-up. Three possible reasons for the neutral outcome in CONSENSUS-II are that it was too short, that only the sort of patient selected for the SAVE trial could benefit, or that ACE inhibition was instituted too early.

The AIRE study randomized patients an average of five days after MI complicated by clinical or radiological signs of heart failure [117]. No specialized tests were required. Only 60% were receiving a diuretic at the time of randomization, indicating that in some patients the heart failure had been mild and/or transient. Beneficial effects on mortality were observed as early as 30 days. This study established that it was feasible on clinical criteria alone to identify a group of patients who had clear benefits with the use of an ACE inhibitor, and that an exercise test was not necessary before initiating therapy. A substudy suggested that about half the patients had an ejection fraction above 40% and therefore would not have been eligible for the SAVE study. The reasons for mortality reduction in AIRE are not yet clear, but recurrent infarction was not reduced significantly. The AIRE study showed that benefit could be achieved within six months, so the duration of CONSENSUS-II was adequate. This suggests that either the time that the ACE inhibitor was given or the selection of the patients was wrong in CONSENSUS-II.

In contrast to SAVE and AIRE, all stable patients with definite MI were eligible to enter the GISSI-III study, and the ACE inhibitor was started within 24 hours of the onset of chest pain. Lisinopril reduced overall mortality, although the incidence of clinical heart failure was not altered [122]. Further reports may identify the reason for the improved prognosis with lisinopril. Benefit was observed in pre-specified subgroups at higher risk after MI, including women and those aged above 70 years. The duration of randomized therapy in GISSI-III was six weeks but follow-up after withdrawal of therapy continued until six months. The early mortality gains made by lisinopril appeared to diminish with time, but as patients with severe ventricular dysfunction or heart failure were likely to receive open-label ACE inhibitor, the data are difficult to interpret. The data could be interpreted as showing that the early benefit of lisinopril is not sustained. Alternatively, they could indicate that the ACE inhibitor must be maintained long term in all patients to sustain or increase benefit. However, the most likely explanation is that the later data were confounded by good clinical practice, that is, the patients who needed an ACE inhibitor received it.

GISSI-III is the first mortality study using an ACE inhibitor to show a benefit with a once-daily dosing regimen. The slow absorption of lisinopril may have prevented very early ACE inhibition, avoiding the problems with hypotension in CONSENSUS-II and ISIS-IV. GISSI-III suggested that selection of patients and duration of follow-up were not the problem with CONSENSUS-II, leaving the third possibility as the most likely reason for the failure of the latter study, that is, the way that the ACE inhibitor was given.

The ISIS-IV study also randomized all infarcts without contraindications and started treatment within 24 hours. It showed that captopril could reduce mortality, although the mechanism by which mortality was reduced remains uncertain. Five percent of patients randomized to placebo had a profound fall in blood pressure requiring termination of treatment, whereas this occurred in 10% of patients randomized to captopril. There were more confirmed infarctions (0.5%, $P < 0.05$) in the captopril group, and it is possible that excessive falls in blood pressure during chest pain precipitated some patients from unstable angina to infarction or increased infarct size [121]. As captopril achieves ACE inhibition more rapidly than other oral ACE inhibitors, there may be hazard involved in the early initiation of captopril. It is notable that the effect of captopril lies between that of lisinopril in GISSI-III and enalapril in CONSENSUS-II. Although captopril 50 mg twice daily may be a less intense and therefore possibly less effective ACE inhibitor regimen than lisinopril 10 mg once daily, enalapril 10 mg twice daily is not. Timing of the onset of ACE inhibition may be the most important difference in these three studies.

Trials using nitrovasodilators

A summary of trials is given in Table 3.19.

In three trials (GISSI-III, ISIS-IV, ESPRIM) nitrovasodilators were not shown to have a significant effect on mortality, though they may be useful in helping relieve peri-infarction angina [122,124]. A non-significant trend was observed for greater benefit when nitrates were used in combination with lisinopril than for lisinopril alone. The results are quite different from what prior meta-analysis had led us to expect [125].

A comparison of placebo and nitroprusside after MI showed no overall difference. However, when patients were stratified according to the delay between the onset of pain to the start of infusion, those patients who had nitroprusside initiated within nine hours of the onset of pain had a significant excess

Nitrovasodilators					
Study	No. of patients Follow-up	Comparison	Recurrent MI	Heart failure	Total mortality Early (late)
Cohn [123] Double-blind	812 21 days and 13 weeks	*Sodium nitroprusside for 48 h* Placebo	ND	ND (pulmonary wedge pressure lower in nitroprusside group)	*16.2%* 18.0% RRR 10% *ns*
GISSI-III 1994 [122] Open label	19 394 6 weeks	*Nitrate patch* Control	*3.1%* 3.2% RRR 3% *ns*	*3.8%* 3.8% *ns*	*6.5%* 6.9% RRR 6% *ns*
ISIS-IV 1994 (unpublished) Double-blind	54 824 35 days	*Oral mononitrate* Placebo	*4.1%* 3.9% R.Excess R 5% *ns*	*17.4%* 17.1% R.Excess R 2% *ns*	*6.98%* 7.22% RRR 3% *ns*
ESPRIM 1993 [124] Double-blind	4017 35 days	*IV + oral molsidomine* Placebo	In-hospital 2.7% 3.3%	In-hospital 7.6% 8.3	*8.4%* *(14.7%)* 8.8% *(14.2%)* RRR 5% *ns*

Table 3.19. MI, myocardial infarction; ND, no data; *ns,* non-significant; RRR, relative risk reduction; R.Excess R, relative excess risk; IV, intravenous.

mortality (24.2% versus 12.7% at 13 weeks; $P=0.025$), while those who started nitroprusside later had a significant improvement in mortality (14.4% versus 22.3%; $P=0.04$). These data suggest that nitrates and probably other hypotensive agents should be used with caution in the first 6–12 hours after MI.

Lipid-lowering by diet or drugs

A summary is shown in Table 3.20 and the results of statin therapy in Table 3.21.

The results from the diet trials are inconclusive, but the Stockholm post-infarction trial showed an unequivocal reduction in all-cause mortality with lipid-lowering drugs. Patients benefited regardless of the level of cholesterol, and the lowering of triglyceride appeared to be more important than reduction in cholesterol. Further confirmation of the benefits of a diet rich in alpha-linolenic acid (the Cretan Mediterranean) is required.

The 4S study showed simvastatin to reduce the risk of further MI, stroke and need for coronary interventions, both following MI and in patients with angina, leading to a reduction in all-cause mortality [131,132]. This confirmed the results of smaller studies with statins in populations with established vascular disease, where trends to improvement were shown [134]. The effects of statins on mortality and morbidity are greater

Lipid-lowering by diet or drugs					
Study	No. of patients Follow-up	Comparison	Non-fatal reinfarction	Stroke	Mortality
DART 1989 [126] Open label	2033 24 months	Dietary fat ↓ *Fatty fish* ↑ Fibre ↓ No advice	3.4% 4.8% 4.0% ND	ND	10.9% *9.3%** 12.1% 9.9%
Singh 1992 [127] Single-blind	505 3 years	*Fat reduction + fruit, nuts + vegetables* Fat reduction only	*14.7%* 23.8% RRR 48% P<0.01	Fatal only *n=1* n=2	*10.3%* 16.8% RRR 59% P<0.01
de Lorgeril [128] Single-blind	605 27 months	Mediterranean diet Usual 'prudent' diet	n=5 (1.7%) n=17 (5.6%) RRR 71% ND	ND	2.6% 6.6% RRR 60% P=0.02
CDP 1975 [129] Double-blind	2840 74 months	*Clofibrate* Nicotinic acid Placebo	*a:13.1%* b: 10.2% c: 13.8% a v c: *ns* b v c: P<0.05	12.3% 8.5% 11.2% *ns*	25.5% 24.4% 25.4% *ns*
Stockholm 1988 [130] Open label	55 5 years	*Clofibrate and nicotinic acid* Control	*12.9%* 18.1% RRR 29% *ns*	*2.2%* 1.8% R.Excess R 2% ns	*21.9%* 29.7% RRR 24% P<0.05

Table 3.20. ND, no data; RRR, relative risk reduction; R.Excess R, relative excess risk. *P<0.05 for advising fatty-fish consumption versus no advice. All other comparisons are non-significant *(ns)*.

Lipid-lowering statin therapy in post-infarct patients					
Study	No. of patients Follow-up Mean age	Comparisons	Non-fatal or fatal MI	Unstable angina	Non-fatal stroke	Mortality
4S 1994 [131,132] Double-blind	4444* 64 months 58 years	Simvastatin 20 mg/day (63%) or 40 mg/day (37%) Placebo	15.9% 22.6% RRR 37% P<0.00001	13.3% 19.9% RRR 11% ns	2.7% 4.3% RRR 30% P=0.024	8.2% 11.5% RRR 30% P=0.0003
CARE 1996 [133]	4159** 60 months 59 years	Pravastatin 40 mg/day Placebo	7.5% 10.0% RRR 25% P<0.01	15.2% 17.3% RRR 13% P=0.07	2.6% 3.8% RRR 31% P=0.03	8.6% 9.4% RRR 9% ns
LIPID 1997 Unpublished	>9000***	Pravastatin 40 mg/day Placebo	Primary endpoint coronary mortality. Study stopped early due to significant benefit in the pravastatin treatment group			

Table 3.21. *About 900 subjects with angina only and 3500 post-MI. Total cholesterol (TC) 5.5–8.0 mmol/l; **TC <6.2 mmol/l; low-density lipoprotein cholesterol (LDL-C) 3.0–4.5 mmol/l; ***TC 4.0–7.0 mmol/l.

than the prognostic benefits of mechanical revascularization for patients with angina—and less expensive over a five-year period [135].

The benefits of simvastatin were shown to occur equally in men and women and in patients with angina and post-MI. Within the cholesterol range studied similar benefits were exerted regardless of the serum cholesterol level. The results of the 4S study have been confirmed in patients with lower cholesterol levels in the CARE [133] and LIPID studies. The WOSCOPS study [136] shows a benefit from statin therapy in populations without established vascular disease but with hyperlipidaemia.

Rehabilitation (exercise-based)

Rehabilitation studies					
Trial	No. of patients Follow-up	Comparisons	Wellbeing	Reinfarction	Mortality
WHO 1983 [137]	2602

3 years | Advice + exercise No special advice | No difference | Non-fatal A < C:8/17* C < A:9/17 | A < C:11/17* C < A:4/17 A = C:2 |
| National Exercise Project 1980 [138] | 651

3 years | Supervised exercise No exercise | Not reported | 5.3% 7.0% RRR 24% ns | 4.6% 7.3% RRR 37% ns |
| Wilhelmsen 1975 [139] | 315

4 years | Supervised exercise Control | Weight, cholesterol, and blood pressure fell in A | 15.8% 17.8% RRR 11% ns | 17.7% 22.3% RRR 24% ns |
| Carson 1982 [140] | 303

1.6 years | Exercise training Control | Less angina (P < 0.05) in A. Return to work similar | 7.3% 6.6% R.Excess R 11% ns | 7.9% 13.8% RRR 43% |
| Ontario 1983 [141] Open label | 733

4 years | Intensive exercise Light exercise | Not reported | 14.2% 13.0% R.Excess R 9% ns | 4.0% 3.7% R.Excess R 8% ns |
| Goble 1991 + Worcester 1993 [142,143] | 308

12 months | Intensive exercise Light exercise | No difference in Q of L scores Exercise performance: A > C | ND | Deaths after entry n = 6 n = 7 |
| EAMI 1993 [144] | 103

6 months | Intensive exercise Control | Exercise performance: A > C No effect on ventricular remodelling | ? None ? None | n = 1 n = 1 |

Table 3.22. *ns*, non-significant; A, active; C, control; RRR, relative risk reduction; R.Excess R, relative excess risk; Q of L, quality of life; ND, no data. *Numbers refer to overall effect in each of 17 centres.

The problem with many of the exercise trials (*see* Table 3.22) is that they compared fairly intensive medical/paramedical supervision 2–3 times per week with relative medical neglect. The studies comparing light and intensive exercise regimens are therefore probably more pertinent to the effects of physical conditioning to outcome after MI, but suggest no specific effect of high-intensity exercise on mortality. None of these studies tests the possibility that even a single exercise test may give reassurance and a psychological boost to the patient who performs well [145,146].

Treatment of diabetes

A summary is given in Table 3.23.

Early studies used retrospective case controls to compare the effects of standard diabetic care with insulin infusion regimens. Standard diabetic care generally constituted the use of a sliding scale of subcutaneous insulin. The effect of insulin infusions on mortality were conflicting. Insulin infusion was attended by a considerable risk of hypoglycaemia and an additional risk of hypokalaemia. More recently the DIGAMI study demonstrated that a combination of insulin and

Treatment of diabetes trials				
Study	No. of patients Follow-up	Comparison	In-hospital heart failure	Total mortality
Gwilt 1984 [147] Retrospective	417 In-hospital	Insulin infusion	47%	33%
		Standard care (usually SC insulin)	35% R.Excess R 34% ns	33% RRR 0% ns
		Non-diabetic control (n = 3 261)		18%
Clark 1985 [148] Retrospective	97 In-hospital	Insulin infusion	34%	16%
		Standard care (usually SC insulin)	36% RRR 6% ns	42% RRR 62% P < 0.05
		Non-diabetic control		~ 13%
DIGAMI 1995 [149] Prospective, randomized	620 1 year	Insulin infusion for 24 hours then SC for 3 months	50%	18.6%
		Standard therapy	48%	26.1% RRR 29% P = 0.027

Table 3.23. SC, subcutaneous; R.Excess R, relative excess risk; RRR, relative risk reduction; *ns*, non-significant.

Glucose–insulin–potassium trials				
Study	No. of patients Follow-up	Comparison	Cardiac arrests (fatal and non-fatal)	Mortality
Mlttra 1965 [150] Open label	170 14 days	SC insulin, oral potassium and glucose for 2 weeks Control	n = 9 n = 17	11.7% 28.2% RRR 59% $P < 0.05$
MRC 1968 [151] Open label	840 28 days	SC insulin, oral potassium and glucose for 2 weeks Control	20.7% 22.6%	23.9% 25.3% RRR 6% ns
Pentecost 1968 [152]	200	IV insulin, potassium and glucose Control	12% 16% RRR ns	15% 16% RRR ns
Rogers 1976 [153] Retrospective	134 In-hospital	IV insulin, potassium and glucose Control	ND	15.7% 29.7% RRR 47% $P < 0.05$

Table 3.24. SC, subcutaneous; RRR, relative risk reduction; ns, non-significant; IV, intravenous; ND, no data.

glucose followed by three months of subcutaneous insulin reduced mortality in patients with diabetes. Most patients were deemed at low risk and had non-insulin-dependent diabetes, but these were the patients who benefited most (52% RRR). Insulin-dependent diabetics and non-insulin-dependent diabetic patients with high risk appeared to obtain less benefit. All the studies are consistent in showing no reduction in post-infarction heart failure in-hospital. Mortality reduction in DIGAMI was not evident until three months. $HbA1_c$ was 7.0% versus 7.5% ($P < 0.01$) at three months in those randomized to insulin versus standard care, respectively. Some 15% of patients developed a hypoglycaemic episode during insulin infusion; 68% of patients were given beta blockers and 48% thrombolytic agents.

Glucose–insulin–potassium (GIK) regimens enjoyed some popularity 20–30 years ago. In view of the DIGAMI results it is of some interest to review this literature. A selection of the better studies is shown in Table 3.24. The results did not show conclusive evidence of benefit in largely non-diabetic populations.

Summary

Early institution of medical care is of paramount importance for optimal management of MI. Thrombolysis, aspirin and access to defibrillation appear highly effective when administered early after MI; class I anti-arrhythmic agents and calcium antagonists should generally be avoided. The timing of initiation and whether ACE inhibitors should be administered to all or only selected patients remain to be settled.

In the longer term, beta blockers (without high ISA) are useful, with verapamil as an alternative. ACE inhibitors should be used in the long term in patients who have had heart failure or have major ventricular dysfunction. Warfarin, but not aspirin, has been shown to improve long-term prognosis. Surgery, angioplasty and exercise rehabilitation have not been proven satisfactorily to reduce mortality, though they may improve symptoms.

Simvastatin has been shown to reduce morbidity and mortality after MI. A considerable amount of the cost of treatment can be recouped by the reduction in need for angioplasty, surgery and readmission with reinfarction. The DIGAMI results suggest that more attention to the management of diabetes after MI is warranted.

References

1. Thurston JGB et al: A controlled investigation into the effects of hyperbaric oxygen on mortality following acute myocardial infarction. Quart J Med 1973, (XLII) 168:751–770.

2. Rawles JM, Kenmure ACF: Controlled trial of oxygen in uncomplicated myocardial infarction. BMJ 1976, 1:1121–1123.

3. Wennerblom B et al: The effect of a mobile coronary care unit on mortality in patients with acute myocardial infarction or cardiac arrest outside hospital. Eur Heart J 1982, 3:504–515.

4. Mathewson SM et al: Mobile coronary care and community mortality from myocardial infarction. Lancet 1985, i:441–443.

5. Dixon RA et al: Diazepam in immediate post-myocardial infarction period. A double-blind trial. Br Heart J 1980, 43:535–540.

6. Pai GR et al: One thousand heart attacks in Grampian: The place of cardiopulmonary resuscitation in general practice. BMJ 1987, 294:352–354.

7. Rivers JT et al: Reinfarction after thrombolytic therapy for acute myocardial infarction followed by conservative management: Incidence and effect of smoking. J Am Coll Cardiol 1990, 16:340–348.

8. GISSI: Effectiveness of intravenous thrombolytic treatment in acute myocardial infarction. Lancet 1986, i:397–402.

9. The International Study Group: In-hospital mortality and clinical course of 20,891 patients with suspected acute myocardial infarction randomised between alteplase and streptokinase with or without heparin. Lancet 1990, 336:71–75.

10. ISIS-2 (Second International Study of Infarct Survival) Collaborative Group: Randomised trial of intravenous streptokinase, oral aspirin, both, or neither among 17,187 cases of suspected acute myocardial infarction: ISIS-2. Lancet 1988, ii:349–360.

11. AIMS Trial Study Group: Long-term effects of intravenous anistreplase in acute myocardial infarction: final report of the AIMS study. Lancet 1990, 335:3–7.

12. Wilcox RG et al: Trial of tissue plasminogen activator for mortality reduction in acute myocardial infarction (ASSET). Lancet 1988, ii:525–533.

13. Wilcox RG et al: Effects of alteplase in acute myocardial infarction: 6-month results from the ASSET study. Lancet 1990, 335:1175–1178.

14. LATE Study Group: Late Assessment of Thrombolytic Efficacy (LATE) study with alteplase 6–24 hours after onset of acute myocardial infarction. Lancet 1993, 342:759–767.

15. EMERAS Collaborative Group: Randomised trial of late thrombolysis in patients with suspected acute myocardial infarction. Lancet 1993, 342:767–772.

16. The European Myocardial Infarction Project Group: Prehospital thrombolytic therapy in patients with suspected acute myocardial infarction. N Engl J Med 1993, 329:383–389.

17. Rawles J, on behalf of the GREAT group: Halving of mortality at 1 year by domiciliary thrombolysis in the Grampian Region Early Anistreplase Trial (GREAT). J Am Coll Cardiol 1994, 23:1–5.

18. GREAT Group: Feasibility, safety and efficacy of domiciliary thrombolysis by general practitioners: Grampian Region Early Anistreplase Trial. BMJ 1992, 305:548–553.

19. Chesebro JH *et al*: Thrombolysis in Myocardial Infarction (TIMI) Trial, phase I: a comparison between intravenous tissue plasminogen activator and intravenous streptokinase. *Circulation* 1987, **76**:142–154.

20. Weaver WD *et al*: Prehospital-initiated vs hospital-initiated thrombolytic therapy. The myocardial infarction triage and intervention trial. *JAMA* 1993, **270**:1211–1216.

21. Longstreth WT *et al*: Myocardial infarction, thromblytic therapy, and stroke. A community based study. *Stroke* 1993, **24**:587–590.

22. Weaver WD *et al*: Effect of age on use of thrombolytic therapy and mortality in acute myocardial infarction. *J Am Coll Cardiol* 1991, **18**:657–662.

23. Fibrinolytic Therapy Triallists (FTT) Collaborative Group: Indications for fibrinolytic therapy in suspected acute myocardial infarction: collaborative overview of early mortality and major morbidity results from all randomised trials of more than 1000 patients. *Lancet* 1994, **343**:311–327.

24. GISSI-2: A factorial randomised trial of alteplase versus streptokinase and heparin versus no heparin among 12,490 patients with acute myocardial infarction. *Lancet* 1990, **336**:65–69.

25. ISIS-3 (Third International Study of Infarct Survival) Collaborative Group: ISIS-3: A randomized comparison of streptokinase vs tissue plasminogen activator vs anistreplase and of aspirin plus heparin vs aspirin alone among 41,299 cases of suspected acute myocardial infarction. *Lancet* 1992, **339**:87–96.

26. The GUSTO Investigators: An international randomized trial comparing four thrombolytic strategies for acute myocardial infarction. *N Engl J Med* 1993, **329**:673–682.

27. Simoons ML *et al*: Thrombolysis with tissue plasminogen activator in acute myocardial infarction; no additional benefit from immediate percutaneous angioplasty. *Lancet* 1988, **i**:197–203.

28. Rogers WJ *et al* for TIMI II-A Investigators: Comparison of immediate invasive delayed invasive and conservative strategies after tissue-type plasminogen activator. *Circulation* 1990, **81**:1457–1475.

29. Williams DO *et al* and TIMI investigators: One-year results of the thrombolysis in myocardial infarction investigation (TIMI) Phase II Trial. *Circulation* 1992, **85**:533–542.

30. SWIFT Trial Study Group: SWIFT trial of delayed elective intervention v. conservative treatment after thrombolysis with anistreplase in acute myocardial infarction. *BMJ* 1991, **302**: 555–560.

31. Ellis SG *et al*: Randomized trial of late elective angioplasty versus conservative management for patients with residual stenoses after thrombolytic treatment of myocardial infarction. *Circulation* 1992, **86**:1400–1406.

32. Topol EJ *et al*: A randomized trial of immediate versus delayed elective angioplasty after intravenous tissue plasminogen activator in acute myocardial infarction. *N Engl J Med* 1987, **317**:582–587.

33. Lee KL *et al*: Multicentre registry of angioplasty therapy for cardiogenic shock. *J Am Coll Cardiol* 1992, **17**:591–603.

34. Hibbard MD *et al*: PTCA in patients with cardiogenic shock. *J Am Coll Cardiol* 1992, **19**: 639–646.

35. O'Neill W *et al*: A prospective randomized clinical trial of intracoronary streptokinase versus coronary angioplasty for acute myocardial infarction. *N Engl J Med* 1986, **314**:812–818.

36. Grines C *et al*: The Primary Angioplasty in Myocardial Infarction Study Group. A comparison of immediate angioplasty with thrombolytic therapy for acute myocardial infarction. *N Engl J Med* 1993, **328**:674–679.

37. Zilstra F *et al*: A comparison of immediate coronary angioplasty with intravenous streptokinase in acute myocardial infarction. *N Engl J Med* 1993, **328**:680–683.

38. Gibbons RJ *et al*: Immediate angioplasty compared with the administration of a thrombolytic agent followed by conservative treatment for myocardial infarction. *N Engl J Med* 1993, **328**:685–691.

39. Vacek JL *et al*: Direct angioplasty versus initial thrombolytic therapy for acute myocardial infarction: long term follow-up and changes in practice pattern. *Am Heart J* 1992, **124**:1411–1417.

40. Jollis JG *et al.*: The relation between the volume of coronary angioplasty procedures at hospitals treating MEDICARE beneficiaries and short-term mortality. *N Engl J Med* 1994, **331**:1625–1629.

41. Lorimer AR *et al* (European Coronary Surgery Bypass Group): The role of early surgery following myocardial infarction. *Br J Clin* 1992, **46**:238–243.

42. Norris RM *et al*: Coronary surgery after recurrent myocardial infarction: progress of a trial comparing surgical with nonsurgical management for asymptomatic patients with advanced coronary disease. *Circulation* 1981, **63**:785–792.

43. Norris RM *et al*: Prognosis after recovery from myocardial infarction: the relative importance of cardiac dilation and coronary stenoses. *Eur Heart J* 1992, **13**:1611–1618.

44. Phillips SJ *et al*: Emergency coronary artery reperfusion: a choice therapy for evolving myocardial infarction. *J Thorac Cardiovasc Surg* 1983, **86**:679–688.

45. Kennedy JW *et al*: Coronary artery bypass graft surgery early after acute myocardial infarction. *Circulation* 1989, **79**:1–73.

46. Bolooki H: Emergency cardiac procedures in patients in cardiogenic shock due to complications of coronary artery disease. *Circulation* 1989, **79** (Suppl I):137–145.

47. Barner HB *et al*: Emergency coronary bypass not associated with preoperative cardiogenic shock in failed angioplasty, after thrombolysis and for acute myocardial infarction. *Circulation* 1989, **79** (Suppl I):152–159.

48. Impact Research Group: International Mexiletine And Placebo Antiarrhythmic Coronary Trial I. Research on arrhythmia and other findings. *J Am Coll Cardiol* 1984, **4**:1148–1163.

49. Berntsen RF, Rasmussen K: Lidocaine to prevent ventricular fibrillation in the prehospital phase of suspected acute myocardial infarction: the North-Norwegian Lidocaine intervention trial. *Am Heart J* 1992, **124**:1478–1483.

50. Campbell RWF *et al*: Prophylaxis of primary ventricular fibrillation with tocainide in acute myocardial infarction. *Br Heart J* 1983, **49**:557–563.

51. Echt DS *et al*: Mortality and morbidity in patients receiving encainide, flecainide, or placebo: the Cardiac Arrhythmia Suppression Trial. *N Engl J Med* 1991, **324**:781–788.

52. The CAST Investigators: Preliminary report: effect of encainide and flecainide on mortality in a randomised trial of arrhythmia suppression after myocardial infarction. *N Engl J Med* 1989, **321**:406–412.

53. The Cardiac Arrhythmia Suppression Trial II Investigators: Effect of the antiarrhythmic agent moricizine on survival after myocardial infarction. *N Engl J Med* 1992, **327**:227–233.

54. Ceremuzynski L *et al*: Effect of amiodarone on mortality after myocardial infarction: a double-blind, placebo-con-

trolled, pilot study. *J Am Coll Cardiol* 1992, **20**:1056–1062.

55. Burkart F *et al*: **Effect of anti-arrhythmic therapy on mortality in survivors of myocardial infarction with asymptomatic complex ventricular arrhythmias: Basel Anti-arrhythmic Study of Infarct Survival (BASIS)**. *J Am Coll Cardiol* 1990, **16**:1711–1718.

56. Pfisterer ME *et al*: **Long-term benefit of one year amiodarone treatment for persistent complex ventricular arrhythmias after myocardial infarction**. *Circulation* 1993, **87**:309–311.

57. Navarro-Lopez F *et al* for the SSSD Investigators: **Comparison of the effects of amiodarone versus metoprolol on the frequency of ventricular arrhythmias and on mortality after acute myocardial infarction**. *Am J Cardiol* 1993, **72**: 1243–1248.

58. Teo KT *et al*: **Effects of prophylactic anti-arrhythmic drug therapy in acute myocardial infarction**. *JAMA* 1993, **270**: 1589–1595.

59. Zarembski DG *et al*: **Empiric long-term amiodarone prophylaxis following myocardial infarction. A meta-analysis.** *Arch Intern Med* 1993, **153**:2661–2667.

60. MacMahon S *et al*: **Effects of prophylactic lidocaine in suspected acute myocardial infarction. An overview of results from the randomized, controlled trials.** *JAMA* 1988, **260**: 1910–1916.

61. Hjalmarson A *et al*: **Effect on mortality of metoprolol in acute myocardial infarction.** *Lancet* 1981, **ii**:823–827.

62. Norris RM *et al*: **Prevention of ventricular fibrillation during acute myocardial infarction by intravenous propranolol.** *Lancet* 1984, **ii**: 883–886.

63. Salathia KS *et al*: **Very early intervention with metoprolol in suspected acute myocardial infarction.** *Eur Heart J* 1985, **6**:190–198.

64. The MIAMI Trial Research Group: **Metoprolol in Acute Myocardial Infarction (MIAMI). A randomised placebo-controlled international trial.** *Eur Heart J* 1985, **6**:199–226.

65. ISIS-1 (First International Study of Infarct Survival) Collaborative Group: **Randomised trial of intravenous atenolol among 16,027 cases of suspected acute myocardial infarction: ISIS-1.** *Lancet* 1981, **ii**:57–65.

66. Roberts R *et al* for the TIMI Investigators: **Immediate versus deferred beta blockade following thrombolytic therapy in patients with acute myocardial infarction. Results of the Thrombolysis In Myocardial Infarction (TIMI) II-B study.** *Circulation* 1991, **83**:422–437.

67. Yusuf S *et al*: **Beta blockade during and after myocardial infarction: an overview of the randomized trials.** *Prog Cardiovasc Dis* 1985, **27**:335–371.

68. The Norwegian Multicenter Study Group: **Timolol-induced reduction in mortality and reinfarction in patients surviving acute myocardial infarction.** *N Engl J Med* 1981, **304**: 801–807.

69. Pedersen TR for the Norwegian Multicenter Study Group: **Six-year follow-up of the Norwegian multicenter study on timolol after acute myocardial infarction.** *N Engl J Med* 1985, **313**:1055–1058.

70. Australian and Swedish Pindolol Study Group: **The effect of pindolol on the two years mortality after complicated myocardial infarction.** *Eur Heart J* 1983, **4**:367–375.

71. Beta-Blocker Heart Attack Trial Research Group: **A randomized trial of propranolol in patients with acute myocardial infarction.** *JAMA* 1983, **250**:2814–2819.

72. Beta Blocker Heart Attack Trial Research Group: **A randomized trial of propranolol in patients with acute myocardial infarction. 1. Mortality results.** *JAMA* 1982, **247**:1707–1714.

73. Julian DG *et al*: **Controlled trial of sotalol for one year after myocardial infarction.** *Lancet* 1982, **i**:1142–1147.

74. European Infarction Study Group (EIS): **A secondary prevention study with slow release oxprenolol after myocardial infarction: morbidity and mortality.** *Eur Heart J* 1984, **5**:189–202.

75. Lopressor Intervention Trial (LIT) Research Group: **The Lopressor Intervention Trial: multicenter study of metoprolol in survivors of acute myocardial infarction.** *Eur Heart J* 1987, **8**:1056–1064.

76. Olsson G *et al*: **Long-term treatment with metoprolol after myocardial infarction: effect on 3 year mortality and morbidity.** *J Am Coll Cardiol* 1985, **5**:1428–1437.

77. Boissel J-P *et al.* (The APSI Investigators): **Secondary prevention after high-risk acute myocardial infarction with low-dose acebutolol.** *Am J Cardiol* 1990, **66**:251–260.

78. Hansen O, Johansson BW: **Benefits of non-selective versus cardioselective beta-blockers in acute myocardial infarction in hypertensive patients.** *J Hypertens* 1993, **11** (Suppl 4):S55–S60.

79. Walker L *et al*: **Effect of nifedipine in the early phase of acute myocardial infarction on enzymatically estimated infarct size and arrhythmias.** *Br Heart J* 1988, **59**:403–410.

80. Wilcox RG *et al* : **Trial of early nifedipine in acute myocardial infarction: the Trent study.** *Br Med J* 1986, **293**:1204–1208.

81. The Israeli Sprint Study Group: **Secondary Prevention Reinfarction Israeli Nifedipine Trial (SPRINT). A randomized intervention trial of Nifedipine in patients with acute myocardial infarction.** *Eur Heart J* 1988, **9**:354–364.

82. Gouldbourt U *et al* for the SPRINT Study Group: **Early administration of nifedipine in suspected acute myocardial infarction. The Secondary Prevention Reinfarction Israel Nifedipine Trial 2 study.** *Arch Intern Med* 1993, **153**:345–352.

83. Gibson R *et al*: **Diltiazem and reinfarction in patients with non-Q wave myocardial infarction.** *N Engl J Med* 1986, **315**:423–429.

84. The Multicenter Diltiazem Postinfarction Trial Research Group: **The effect of diltiazem on mortality and reinfarction after myocardial infarction.** *N Engl J Med* 1988, **319**:385–392.

85. The Danish Study Group on Verapamil in Myocardial Infarction: **Verapamil in acute myocardial infarction.** *Eur Heart J* 1984, **5**: 516–528.

86. The Danish Study Group on Verapamil in Myocardial Infarction: **Effect of verapamil on mortality and major events after acute myocardial infarction (The Danish Verapamil Infarction Trial II – Davit II).** *Am J Cardiol* 1990, **66**:779–785.

87. Yusuf S *et al*: **Update of effects of calcium antagonists in myocardial infarction or angina in light of the second Danish verapamil trial (DAVIT-II) and other recent studies.** *Am J Cardiol* 1991, **67**:1295–1297.

88. The RISK Group: **Risk of myocardial infarction and death during treatment with low dose aspirin and intravenous heparin in men with unstable coronary artery disease.** *Lancet* 1990, **336**:827–830.

89. Elwood PC *et al*: **A randomized controlled trial of acetyl salicylic acid in the secondary prevention of mortality from myocardial infarction.** *BMJ* 1974, **308**:436–441.

90. Elwood PC, Sweetnam PM: **Aspirin and secondary mortality after myocardial infarction.** *Lancet* 1979, **ii**:1313–1315.

91. The Coronary Drug Project Research Group: **Aspirin in coronary heart disease.** *Circulation* 1980, **62** (Suppl V):59–62.

92. Aspirin Myocardial Infarction Study Research Group: **A randomized, controlled trial of aspirin in persons recovered from myocardial infarction.** *JAMA* 1980, **243**:661–668.

93. The Aspirin Myocardial Infarction Study Reseach Group: **The Aspirin Myocardial Infarction Study: final results.** *Circulation* 1980, **62** (Suppl V):79–83.

94. The Persantine-Aspirin Reinfarction Study (PARIS) Research Group: **The Persantine-Aspirin Reinfarction Study.** *Circulation* 1980, **62** (Suppl V):85–87.

95. The Persantine-Aspirin Reinfarction Study (PARIS) Research Group: **Persantine and aspirin in coronary heart disease.** *Circulation* 1980, **62**:449–462.

96. Klimt CR *et al*: **Persantine-Aspirin Reinfarction Study. Part II. Secondary coronary prevention with persantine and aspirin.** *J Am Coll Cardiol* 1987, **7**:251–269.

97. Antiplatelet Trialists' Collaboration: **Secondary prevention of vascular disease by prolonged antiplatelet treatment.** *BMJ* 1988, **296**:320–331.

98. Antiplatelet Trialists' Collaboration: **Collaborative overview of randomised trials of antiplatelet therapy. I. Prevention of death, myocardial infarction, and stroke by prolonged antiplatelet therapy in various categories of patients.** *BMJ* 1994, **308**:81–106.

99. Breddin K *et al*: **The German-Austrian Aspirin Trial: a comparison of acetylsalicylic acid, placebo and phenprocoumon in secondary prevention of myocardial infarction.** *Circulation* 1980, **62** (Suppl V):63–71.

100. The EPSIM Research Group: **A controlled comparison of aspirin and oral anticoagulants in prevention of death after myocardial infarction.** *N Engl J Med* 1982, **307**:702–709.

101. Working Party on Anticoagulant Therapy in Coronary Thrombosis to the Medical Research Council: **Assessment of short-term anticoagulant administration after cardiac infarction.** *BMJ* 1969, **1**:335–341.

102. Veterans Administration Cooperative Clinical Trial: **Anticoagulants in acute myocardial infarction.** *JAMA* 1973, **225**:724–729.

103. Second Report of the Working Party on Anticoagulant Therapy in Coronary Thrombosis to the Medical Research Council: **An assessment of long-term anticoagulant administration after cardiac infarction.** *BMJ* 1964, **2**:837–843.

104. Ebert RV *et al* (Veterans Administration Cooperative Study): **Long-term anticoagulant therapy after myocardial infarction.** *JAMA* 1969, **207**:2263–2267.

105. Report of Sixty Plus Reinfarction Study Research Group: **A double-blind trial to assess long-term oral anticoagulant therapy in elderly patients after myocardial infarction.** *Lancet* 1980, **ii**:989–994.

106. Smith P *et al*: **The effect of warfarin on mortality and reinfarction after myocardial infarction.** *N Engl J Med* 1990, **323**:147–151.

107. ASPECT Research Group (Anticoagulants in the Secondary Prevention of Events in Coronary Thrombosis): **Effect of long-term oral anticoagulant treatment on mortality and cardiovascular morbidity after myocardial infarction.** *Lancet* 1994, **343**:499–503.

108. The SCATI Group: **Randomised controlled trial of subcutaneous calcium-heparin in acute myocardial infarction.** *Lancet* 1989, **ii**: 182–186.

109. Serneri GGN *et al* (Italian Study Group on Prevention of Myocardial Reinfarction by Low Dose Heparin): **Effectiveness of low-dose heparin in prevention of myocardial reinfarction.** *Lancet* 1987, **i**:937–942.

110. Serneri GGN: **Long-term follow-up of heparin to prevent myocardial infarction** [Letter]. *Lancet* 1993, **342**:48.

111. Woods K *et al*: **Intravenous magnesium sulphate in suspected acute myocardial infarction: results of the second Leicester Intravenous Magnesium Intervention Trial (LIMIT-2).** *Lancet* 1992, **339**:1553–1558.

112. Woods KL, Fletcher S: **Long-term outcome after intravenous magnesium sulphate in suspected acute myocardial infarction: the second Leicester Intravenous Magnesium Intervention Trial (LIMIT-2).** *Lancet* 1994, **343**:807–809, 816–819.

113. Teo K *et al*: **Effects of intravenous magnesium in suspected acute myocardial infarction: overview of randomised trials.** *BMJ* 1991, **303**:1499–1503.

114. Galloe AM *et al.*: **Influence of oral magnesioum supplementation on cardiac events among survivors of an acute myocardial infarction.** *BMJ* 1993, **307**:585–587.

115. Swedberg K *et al*: **Effects of the early administration of enalapril on mortality in patients with acute myocardial infarction.** *N Engl J Med* 1992, **327**:678–684.

116. Pfeffer MA *et al*: **Effect of captopril on mortality and morbidity in patients with left ventricular dysfunction after myocardial infarction.** *N Engl J Med* 1992, **327**:669–677.

117. The Acute Infarction Ramipril Efficacy (AIRE) Study Investigators: **Effect of ramipril on mortality and morbidity of survivors of acute myocardial infarction with clinical evidence of heart failure.** *Lancet* 1993, **342**:821–828.

118. Foy SG *et al.*: **Comparison of enalapril versus captopril on left ventricular function and survival three months after acute myocardial infarction (The 'PRACTICAL' Study).** *Am J Cardiol* 1994, **73**:1180–1186.

119. Amrosioni E, Borghi C, Magnani B: **The effect of the angiotensin-converting-enzyme inhibitor zofenopril on mortality and morbidity after myocardial infarction.** *N Engl J Med* 1995, **332**:80–85.

120. The TRACE Study Group: **The Trandolapril Cardiac Evaluation (TRACE) Study: rationale, design and baseline characteristics of the screened population.** *Am J Cardiol* 1994, **73**:40C–50C.

121. Cleland JGF: **ACE inhibitors for myocardial infarction: how should they be used?** *Eur Heart J* 1995, **16**:153–159.

122. GISSI-III: **Effects of lisinopril and transdermal glyceryl trinitrate singly and together on 6-week mortality and ventricular function after acute myocardial infarction.** *Lancet* 1994, **343**:1115–1122.

123. Cohn JN *et al.*: **Effect of short-term infusion of sodium nitroprusside on mortality rate in acute myocardial infarction complicated by left ventricular failure.** *N Engl J Med* 1982, **301**:1129–1135.

124. The ESPRIM Trial: **Short-term treatment of acute myocardial infarction with molsidomine.** *Lancet* 1994, **344**:91–97.

125. Yusuf S *et al*: **Effect of intravenous nitrates on mortality in acute myocardial infarction: an overview of the randomised trials.** *Lancet* 1988, **i**:1088–1092.

126. Burr ML *et al*: **Effects of changes in fat, fish and fibre intakes on death and myocardial reinfarction: diet and reinfarction trial (DART).** *Lancet* 1989, **ii**:757–761.

127. Singh RB *et al*: **Randomised controlled trial of cardioprotective diet in patients with recent acute myocardial infarction: results of one year follow up.** *BMJ* 1992, **304**:1015–1019.

128. de Lorgeril M *et al.*: **Mediterranean alpha-linoleic acid-rich diet in secondary prevention of coronary heart disease.** *Lancet* 1994, **343**:1454–1459.

129. The Coronary Drug Project Research Group: **Clofibrate and niacin in coronary heart disease.** *JAMA* 1975, **231**:360–381.

130. Carlson LA, Rosenhamer G: **Reduction of mortality in the Stockholm Ischaemic Heart Disease Secondary**

Prevention Study by combined treatment with clofibrate and nicotinic acid. *Acta Med Scand* 1988, **223**: 405–418.

131. Scandinavian Simvastatin Survival Study Group: **Randomised trial of cholesterol lowering in 4444 patients with coronary artery disease: the Scandinavian Simvastatin Survival Study (4S).** *Lancet* 1994, **344**:1383–1389.

132. Pedersen WR: **Baseline serum cholesterol and treatment effect in the Scandinavian Simvastatin Survival Study.** *Lancet* 1995, **345**:1274–1275.

133. Sacks FM, Pfeffer MA, Moye LA, *et al.*: **The effect of pravastatin on coronary events after myocardial infarction in patients with average cholesterol levels.** *N Engl J Med* 1996, **335**:1001–1009.

134. Cleland JGF: **Clinical trials in stable and unstable angina.** In Cleland JGF (ed): *Asymptomatic Coronary Artery Disease and Angina.* London: Science Press; 1996, pp 62–100.

135. Cleland JGF, Walker A: **Is medical treatment for angina the mos cost effective option?** *Eur Heart J* 1997, **18**:b35–b42.

136. Shepherd J, Cobbe SM, Ford I, *et al.* for the West of Scotland Coronary Prevention Study Group: **Prevention of coronary heart disease with pravastatin in men with hypercholesterolaemia.** *N Engl J Med* 1995, **333**:1301–1307.

137. Lamm G *et al*: **Rehabilitation and secondary prevention of patients after acute myocardial infarction.** *Adv Cardiol* 1982, **31**: 107–111.

138. Shaw LW (for staff of National Exercise and Heart Disease Project): **Effects of a prescribed supervised exercise program on mortality and cardiovascular morbidity in patients after a myocardial infarction.** *Am J Cardiol* 1981, **48**:39–45.

139. Wilhelmsen L *et al*: **A controlled trial of physical training after myocardial infarction.** *Prev Med* 1975, **4**:491–508.

140. Carson P *et al*: **Exercise after myocardial infarction: a controlled trial.** *J R Coll Phys Lond* 1982, **16**:147–151.

141. Rechnitzer P *et al*: **Relation of exercise to the recurrence rate of myocardial infarction in men. Ontario Exercise–Heart Collaborative Study.** *Am J Cardiol* 1983, **51**:65–69.

142. Goble AJ *et al*: **Effect of early programmes of high and low intensity exercise on physical performance after transmural acute myocardial infarction.** *Br Heart J* 1991, **65**:126–131.

143. Worcester MC *et al*: **Early programmes of high and low intensity exercise and quality of life after acute myocardial infarction.** *BMJ* 1993, **307**:1244.

144. Giannuzzi P *et al*: **Long-term physical training and left ventricular remodeling after anterior myocardial infarction: results of the exercise in anterior myocardial infarction (EAMI) trial.** *J Am Coll Cardiol* 1993, **22**:1821–1829.

145. Oldridge NB *et al*: **Cardiac rehabilitation after myocardial infarction. Combined experience of randomized clinical trials.** *JAMA* 1988, **260**:945–949.

146. O'Connor GT *et al*: **An overview of randomized trials of rehabilitation with exercise after myocardial infarction.** *Circulation* 1989, **80**:234–244.

147. Gwilt DJ *et al.*: **Effect of intravenous infusion on mortality among diabetic patients after myocardial infarction.** *Br Heart J* 1984, **51**:626–630.

148. Clark RS *et al.*: **Effect of intravenous infusion of insulin in diabetics with acute myocardial infarction.** *Br Med J Clin Res Ed* 1985, **291**:303–305.

149. Malmberg *et al.*: **Diabets Insulin Glucose Acute Myocardial Infarction (DIGAMI) Study.** (*J Am Coll Cardiol*, in press 1995).

150. Mittra B: **Potassium, glucose and insulin in treatment of myocardial infarction.** *Lancet* 1965, **ii**: 607–609.

151. MRC Working Party in the Treatment on Myocardial Infarction: **Potassium, glucose and insulin treatment for acute myocardial infarction.** *Lancet* 1968, **ii**:1355–1360.

152. Pentecost BL, Mayne NMC, Lamb P: **Controlled trial of intravenous glucose potassium and insulin in acute myocardial infarction.** *Lancet* 1968, **I**:946–948.

153. Rogers WJ *et al.*: **Reduction of hospital mortality rate of acute myocardial infarction with glucose-insulin potassium infusion.** *Am Heart J* 1976, **92**:441–454.

CHAPTER 4

Management in perspective

John GF Cleland

A general policy for the management of patients after MI is shown in Table 4.1.

Management of patients post-MI				
	Day 1	Day 2 until discharge	Assessments at weeks 4–6	Long-term
Investigation	Confirm infarction (ECG + enzymes) Lipids Urea + electrolytes Full blood count	Clinical observation Consider angiography if angina at rest or slight exertion	Measure LV function Consider angiography if +ve ETT* at < 6 min	LV function in selected individuals Risk factors for ischaemic heart disease
Rehabilitation and investigation		ETT* (symptom limited)	ETT* (symptom limited)	Exercise programme in individuals requiring support
Treatment	Analgesia Defibrillator access Aspirin Early thrombolysis Beta blocker Nitrate	Aspirin Beta blocker ACE inhibitor	Risk factors for ischaemic heart disease	Good LV function, Low-risk ETT: Aspirin + statin** Good LV function, Non-low-risk ETT: Aspirin + statin** Beta blocker Poor LV function: Warfarin + statin** Beta blocker (if tolerated) ACE inhibitor

Table 4.1. MI, myocardial infarction; ECG, electrocardiogram; LV, left ventricular; ETT, exercise tolerance test; ACE, angiotensin-converting enzyme. *May be omitted if resources are limited; **recommended for all MIs if cholesterol > 5.6 mmol/l despite a trial diet of six months.

The first 24 hours

The mortality within the first 24 hours after MI remains high. One-half or more of all deaths in the first month occur before patients reach hospital.

Investigations

These are largely directed at confirming MI and include the 12-lead ECG and cardiac enzymes or measurement of myoglobin or troponin. ECG monitoring to detect arrhythmias is standard, although it is unclear whether prophylaxis of arrhythmias is useful. Routine biochemical tests should be carried out to detect hypokalaemia which may require correction. Routine haematology screening is useful in excluding concomitant disease. Lipids should be checked early because plasma cholesterol falls in the aftermath of MI and may lead to failure to detect hyperlipidaemia. A chest radiogram is not essential at this stage and, unless it can be obtained in the safety of the CCU, need not be performed unless there is diagnostic doubt about the cause of chest pain or breathlessness. Invasive monitoring, echocardiography or radionuclide techniques for imaging the ventricle or infarcted area are not necessary unless the patient is in haemodynamic difficulties.

Treatment
Opiate analgesia
The early studies comparing mobile CCUs and hospital treatment had little more to offer than general care, oxygen, analgesia, defibrillation and anti-arrhythmic therapy. Despite this, they showed substantial reductions in mortality with early treatment. Prophylactic anti-arrhythmic therapy and oxygen do not appear effective, while the number of lives saved by defibrillation does not seem great enough to account for the difference. This indirect evidence suggests that adequate analgesia, which reduces pain and sympathetic activity, may have a substantial impact on mortality. Care must be exercised in those patients with chronic respiratory disease. Small doses of diamorphine (2.5 mg), repeated as required, are suggested. Intravenous metoclopramide (10 mg) should be given to prevent nausea and vomiting.
- Lives saved (predicted) in the first month per thousand patients treated: 100+.

Anti-thrombotic strategy
The evidence in favour of giving aspirin as soon as possible (160 mg enteric-coated was used in ISIS-II)) is now overwhelming. The evidence in favour of heparin or warfarin at this stage is less robust.
- Lives saved in the first month per thousand patients treated: 25 (also four strokes per thousand and 15 reinfarctions per thousand treated). Benefit maintained, but not increasing, with long-term follow-up.

Defibrillation
Provision should be made to get the patient to an area where he or she can be defibrillated as quickly as possible or get a defibrillator to the patient. Local circumstances will dictate whether this is performed by the GP, paramedics or hospital.
- Lives saved in the first month per thousand patients treated: 40–50 (ten per thousand out of hospital given adequate facilities).

Thrombolysis
This should be given as quickly as possible. Again local circumstances will dictate who should give thrombolysis and where. An ECG and the clinical history alone suf-

General contraindications to thrombolysis	
Absolute	**Relative**
• Active source of bleeding that cannot be controlled (includes gastrointestinal and heavy vaginal bleeding)	• Hypertension
• Vascular surgery or major trauma within previous 10 days	• Any previous stroke
• Stroke or central nervous system surgery within previous 2 months	• Active or recent peptic ulcer (not bleeding)
• Subclavian line	
• Recent traumatic cardiopulmonary resuscitation	• Risk of bleeding from a site that can be controlled (e.g. femoral artery puncture)
• Known bleeding diathesis	
• Pregnancy	
• Known intracranial neoplasm or aneurysm	

Table 4.2.

fice to decide who should receive thrombolysis. Absolute and relative contraindications are listed in Table 4.2.

Which thrombolytic? Streptokinase is effective and inexpensive but is not user-friendly, either in the community or possibly the casualty department, because of the need to set up an infusion. It may cause hypotension, although this is usually transient. It is advisable to administer streptokinase to a patient only once in their lifetime, as on the second occasion allergic reactions may occur. Even if this does not happen, antibodies that neutralize the action of streptokinase may persist for years.

APSAC is more convenient and more expensive. There is a slightly higher risk of hypotension than with either of the other agents. Ideally, as with streptokinase, APSAC should be given only once in a lifetime. Contraindications to APSAC are given in Table 4.3.

tPA is the agent of choice for patients requiring a thrombolytic the second time

Specific contraindications to streptokinase or APSAC	
Absolute	**Relative**
Allergy to streptokinase	Hypotension
Administration of either in past 12 months	Administration of either ever before

Table 4.3. APSAC, anisoylated plasminogen-streptokinase activator complex.

round, or in patients who develop an allergic reaction to one of the above agents. It may be the first choice in those patients who are already hypotensive. Tissue-type plasminogen activator may achieve more rapid thrombolysis, thus supporting its use in younger patients with large anterior infarcts presenting within the first 2–3 hours after infarction to preserve ventricular function better, and thereby improve long-term prognosis. It is relatively contraindicated in older patients and in those with hypertension as it is associated with more strokes than use of streptokinase or APSAC. It is not clear whether heparin needs to be given with tPA, as suggested in the GUSTO trial.

• The use of combinations of thrombolytic agents cannot be advocated at present.

Late thrombolysis? The benefits of thrombolysis greatly outweigh the risks in the first 12 hours. After 12 hours the risks and benefits of thrombolysis are more evenly balanced, and it may be wise to confine treatment to younger patients and anterior or large infero-posterior infarcts.

• Lives saved per thousand patients treated in the first month: 25.
• Lives saved per thousand patients treated in the first year: 30.

Beta blockers

A definite benefit with propranolol and atenolol in the first 24 hours was shown in studies before the advent of thrombolysis. Non-selective agents (that may reduce hypokalaemia caused by high sympathetic activity more effectively) may be superior to selective agents in reducing mortality. Early intravenous use in the community may reduce pre-hospital mortality. It remains to be proven whether intravenous beta blockade in hospital is still necessary with the advent of thrombolysis. However, as beta blockers probably slow the rate of myocardial necrosis and possibly reduce cardiac rupture, which is increased by late thrombolysis, a beneficial interaction with thrombolytic agents might be expected.

There are therefore good reasons for administering intravenous beta blockers to patients who have a contraindication to thrombolysis (*see* Table 4.4) or to those who receive thrombolysis late. Overall, early beta blockade does no harm, and it may be a simpler policy to give it to all patients in the absence of contraindications. Whether it is necessary to give it intravenously or orally in the first 24 hours has not been tested.

• Lives saved per thousand patients treated in the first week: 5.
• Lives saved per thousand patients treated for one week at one year: 15.

ACE inhibitors

Although much of the left ventricular dilatation that occurs after MI does so in the first 24 hours, this may be a necessary and indeed beneficial response to the infarct itself. Larger infarcts may necessitate greater dilatation to maintain stroke

Contraindications to beta blockers	
Absolute	**Relative**
Asthma	Overt heart failure other than pulmonary oedema
Pulmonary oedema	Bradycardia/heart block
	Hypotension
	Severe peripheral vascular disease

Table 4.4. Overall, beta blockade has been shown to be harmless unless any of the above contra-indications exist.

volume and prevent an excessive rise in filling pressures. Thus, although greater dilatation is associated with a worse prognosis, this may reflect the size of the infarct at this stage and not ventricular maladaptation.

The CONSENSUS-II study indicated that very early introduction of an ACE inhibitor was potentially harmful. The ISIS-IV and GISSI-III studies indicate that slightly later introduction improves survival. More patients given captopril developed infarction in ISIS-IV, possibly due to the induction of hypotension leading to coronary occlusion in patients with unstable angina. This suggests either that an ACE inhibitor with a slow onset of action (such as lisinopril) should be used or that the introduction of the ACE inhibitor should be delayed beyond the first 24 hours. The latter is my preferred policy.

- Lives saved per thousand patients treated in the first six weeks: 8 (assuming optimal timing as discussed above).
- Lives saved per thousand treated in the first year: about 25.

Magnesium
The role of magnesium remains uncertain. No recommendation for routine use can be made at present. Magnesium was given some time after thrombolysis in ISIS-IV but before thrombolysis in LIMIT-II. A study comparing simultaneous administration of magnesium and thrombolytic compared with thrombolytic alone is required.

Nitrates
Nitrates have a valuable role in relieving the pain of unstable angina, in reducing blood pressure in hypertensive patients and for the treatment of pulmonary oedema after MI. The ISIS-IV trial also indicates that nitrates may reduce mortality in the first 24 hours, although no long-term benefit was apparent. There was a trend towards greater reduction in mortality in those treated with transdermal nitrates and lisinopril in GISSI-III and almost all of this difference could be attributed to a reduction in mortality among those who developed hypotension

with lisinopril, presumably in the early post-infarction period. The use of a single buccal nitrate in the immediate post-infarction period would appear simple and to have some merit for these reasons. Nitrates may induce severe hypotension and even shock if filling pressures are reduced excessively.

Treatment of diabetes

The DIGAMI protocol should be followed wherever possible (Table. 4.5).

DIGAMI insulin protocol	
Infusate	500 ml 5% glucose with 80 IU soluble insulin
Infusion	Initially 30 ml/hour. Adjust according to target blood glucose. Reduce rate of infusion to 15 ml/hour after 10 pm if blood glucose < 11 mmol/l
Target blood glucose	7–10 mmol/l
Blood glucose monitoring	Hourly unless infusion rate stable, in which case every 2 hours
Blood glucose > 15 mmol/l	Give 8 IU of insulin as intravenous bolus and increase infusion rate by 6 ml/hour
Blood glucose 11–15 mmol/l	Increase infusion rate by 3 ml/hour
Blood glucose 7–11 mmol/l	No change
Blood glucose 4–7 mmol/l	Reduce infusion rate by 3 ml/hour
Blood glucose < 4 mmol/l	Stop infusion. Administer glucose if necessary
At 24 h	Convert to SC insulin
Soluble insulin	Three times a day before meals
Medium long-acting	Evening dose

Table 4.5. IU, international unit; SC, subcutaneous; DIGAMI, Diabetic patients receiving Insulin-Glucose infusion during Acute Myocardial Infarction.

Day two to six weeks

Investigations

In addition to routine clinical care, some specialized investigations may be required. The need for investigation depends on treatment policy and how accurate a prediction of prognosis is required. Although many investigations have been shown to predict outcome, few are of definite use in making clinical decisions.

The timing of these investigations may need to be adapted to the individual unit's circumstances, but a broad policy needs to be established if problems are to be anticipated and prevented rather than the physician reacting to a series of medical crises.

Investigations performed too late may fail to identify patients requiring early intervention. Those performed too early may identify patients with a poorer prognosis but who cannot benefit from early intervention (e.g., early coronary angiography may identify a patient with left main coronary disease who would benefit from surgery but in whom it is advisable to wait until the infarct scar has stabilized before operating). Early investigation will not always identify some high-risk patients (e.g., the patient in whom LV dilatation occurs late). Early investigation may also mean that the patient may have to be re-investigated if the infarct extends or other problems occur. Ventricular function may improve as "stunned" myocardium recovers. Early investigation may inappropriately identify these patients' need for therapy. It is also often more cost-efficient to organize investigations with a 3–6-week waiting list.

If it is the policy to treat all patients after MI with aspirin, beta blocker and an ACE inhibitor, then no further investigation is necessary at this stage, in the absence of angina at rest or slight exertion. If a selective policy on ACE inhibitor use is adopted, then ventricular function needs to be quantified. If a selective policy on beta blockers is adopted, then exercise testing and measurements of ventricular function can identify low-risk groups where the benefits of beta blockade will be minimal. If angina occurs at rest or slight exertion, then the patient may be observed in hospital in the hope that symptoms will settle on medical therapy (as will usually occur) or referred for coronary arteriography (left ventricular angiography should be avoided as it may dislodge the thrombus).

Treatment
Anti-thrombotic strategy
Aspirin remains the drug of choice, but in large anterior infarcts the risk of embolic stroke is high, and there are arguments for using heparin and/or warfarin. For patients with complications that require prolonged bed rest, subcutaneous heparin for the prophylaxis of deep venous thrombosis is required.

Beta blockers
Two policies may be adopted:
- Start all patients on a beta blocker before discharge.
- Assess ventricular function and exercise performance. If results are satisfactory (i.e. no angina or ST segment depression on a symptom-limited test), the patient's risk is low and it is unlikely that beta blockers will improve outcome.

The first option is preferred because this conforms most closely to the clinical trials.

Calcium antagonists

Verapamil is the calcium antagonist of choice in patients in whom a beta blocker is contraindicated because of respiratory or peripheral vascular disease.

Verapamil should be avoided in patients with heart failure or with higher degrees of heart block. Constipation is much less of a problem with slow-release preparations. The evidence in favour of diltiazem is less striking and nifedipine may be harmful.

ACE inhibitors

The ISIS-IV and GISSI-III studies showed that ACE inhibitors can reduce mortality in the first six weeks after MI when given to all patients, and did not identify any subgroup of patients who did not benefit.

The AIRE study suggested even greater benefits (in terms of lives saved) in the first 30 days after infarction, if only patients with clinical evidence of failure were treated, treatment being started 2–3 days after infarction. The SAVE study did not show any survival benefit until after the first year!

This suggests three options:

• Treat all patients with an ACE inhibitor.
• Treat only patients with clinical or radiological evidence of heart failure.
• Assess ventricular function and treat patients with marked dysfunction or heart failure.

Although those patients with clinical or radiological evidence of heart failure will benefit most from ACE inhibition, substantial benefit may be obtained in other patients. Early measurement of ventricular function may over- or underestimate the severity of chronic ventricular dysfunction and, if resources limit the number of echocardiograms that can be done, it may be better to wait until ventricular function has stabilized in order to judge the need for long-term therapy. It is therefore suggested that all patients are treated with an ACE inhibitor initially.

Nitrates

On current evidence nitrates should not be used beyond the acute period.

Surgery and PTCA

Unless the patient has angina that cannot be controlled by medical therapy, or major haemodynamic upset caused by a ventricular septal defect or mitral regurgitation, surgery should be avoided until the infarct scar has healed.

PTCA after thrombolysis for MI has consistently been shown to be ineffective in large trials.

The morphology of the ruptured plaque may change dramatically in the weeks following an infarction, and the severity of the infarct-related stenosis usually becomes less severe.

For these reasons, angiography should be avoided if possible in the first six weeks after infarction.

Rehabilitation

Rehabilitation, although reassuring for the patient, makes little difference to physical aspects of the disease and is not a priority area at this stage. However, a pre-discharge exercise test, if satisfactory, is very reassuring for the patient.

From six weeks

Investigations

All patients should have ventricular function measured within the first six weeks. If resources are limited, then imaging at about six weeks is probably optimal because:

• ventricular damage and recovery should have stabilized
• a decision on whether to continue long-term ACE inhibition has to be made.

There is considerable evidence to support exercise testing, but the ideal timing is controversial and there are major advantages in carrying out both early and late testing (*see* Table. 4.6).

Early and late exercise testing			
Advantages of early testing	**Disadvantages of early testing**	**Advantages of late testing**	**Disadvantages of late testing**
Psychological reassurance before discharge	No evidence that the adverse prognosis indicated by a positive test can be altered by specific therapy	Positive test better predictor of long-term angina	May miss early events
Detect high-risk patients early	Surgery early post-infarction relatively contraindicated	No contraindication to surgery if needed on the basis of a strongly positive test and further investigations	Little evidence that the adverse prognosis indicated by a positive test can be altered by specific therapy
Low-risk patients on basis of ETT may not need beta blocker	Poor correlation between early and late tests; early testing poor predictor of long-term angina	Helps decide whether patient needs long-term beta blocker	
	Highest risk group are those deemed unable to exercise		

Table 4.6. ETT, exercise tolerance test.

If resources are limited then a test at six weeks probably provides more information that is likely to alter clinical decisions.

Coronary angiography
This should be considered in patients with limiting angina not responding to medical therapy or if the side effects of medical treatment are major. Patients with a positive low-level exercise test (i.e. 1 mm ST depression at six minutes on a Bruce protocol) should be considered for investigation if they are candidates for intervention.

Treatment
Antithrombotic strategy
The evidence in favour of long-term prophylaxis with aspirin after MI is lacking. Although meta-analysis has suggested long-term benefit in terms of mortality, the findings are of marginal statistical significance despite the large number of patients. It should be remembered that before the ISIS-IV study meta-analysis of magnesium and nitrate studies had suggested far more powerful beneficial effects than the modest effect of aspirin long term. It is curious that despite an apparent reduction in reinfarction, aspirin has not effectively reduced mortality or the incidence of heart failure in the long term. It is possible that aspirin increases the proportion of silent infarctions, and, indeed, a trend to an increase in sudden death (perhaps reflecting silent infarction) is a consistent feature of the long-term aspirin studies.

The evidence in favour of long-term warfarin is stronger but, with only one of the three largest studies reporting a clear-cut reduction in mortality, further evaluation is required. However, for patients at high risk of recurrent infarction or death the case for warfarin is strong.

In patients with heart failure the long-term trials show a non-significant excess mortality with aspirin. There are no data with warfarin. The effects of warfarin, aspirin and no antithrombotic therapy are currently being studied in a large study (WASH).

Beta blockers/verapamil
If, after assessment of ventricular function and exercise performance, the patient's prognosis is considered to be excellent (i.e., well preserved ventricular function and no angina or ST segment depression on a symptom-limited test), it is justified to consider stopping these treatments. However, it is not clear whether this commits the cardiologist to repeat (possibly annual) testing in order to ensure that the patient remains at low risk. It is perfectly reasonable if the patient is free of troublesome side effects to continue these treatments indefinitely, in which case there is no need for repeat testing.

ACE inhibitors
If ventricular function is well preserved and the patient has never had evidence of heart failure the ACE inhibitor may be stopped. Unless a further major ischaemic insult takes place, well preserved ventricular function is usually stable and repeat

testing is not required (some might argue for repeat testing at 5–10-year intervals although evidence is lacking). Some patients exhibit features of heart failure after infarction but appear to have well preserved ventricular function. In view of the outstanding results of the AIRE study, it is probably best to continue these patients on an ACE inhibitor indefinitely.

Surgery and PTCA
These interventions should be considered in patients with angina which is not controlled by medical therapy or where the side effects of medical treatment are major. In patients who have required angiography, surgery may be necessary in those with severe multi-vessel disease or left main coronary stenosis.

Rehabilitation
Patients who are having difficulty coming to terms with the infarction should be referred for counselling and possibly physical rehabilitation. If resources are available a light-exercise rehabilitation programme appears as useful as a more intense programme.

Risk-factor management
The patient's risk factors require major reappraisal.

Has the patient started *smoking* again? Stopping smoking will prevent about 60 reinfarctions in the first year [1].

Blood pressure should be controlled. In view of the positive outcome in post-infarction trials, beta blockers, ACE inhibitors and verapamil are indicated. Hypertension trials have shown that thiazides reduce MI; therefore thiazides are indicated. There is no evidence to support the use of dihydropyridine calcium antagonists (e.g., nifedipine, amlodipine), diltiazem or alpha blockers, as yet.

Treatment of *hyperlipidaemia* is now accepted. The patient should be advised to include more fatty fish and more fruit, nuts and vegetables in their diet. There is no evidence in post-infarction trials that reducing animal fats is useful but it is probably appropriate to follow such advice as for patients with hyperlipidaemia and known vascular disease. Patients with blood cholesterol >5.6mmol/l despite a lipid-lowering diet should receive drug therapy. A statin is the simplest and most effective treatment. Those who wish to follow the published evidence should try diet for the first six months. The efficacy, and indeed safety, of early treatment have not been established.

Despite a variety of guidelines there is no evidence to substantiate what level of cholesterol should be treated after MI. Children have a cholesterol of about 3–4 mmol/l [2] — perhaps this is the safest level? Patients with diabetes should receive subcutaneous insulin for three months [3], regardless of whether they are normally insulin- dependent or not.

Management of clinical complications
of myocardial infarction

Rest angina

Chest pain recurring at rest more than 24 hours after the onset of infarction is omi-
nous and probably more common since the advent of thrombolysis. Between 20 and
40% of patients with recurrent chest pain more than 24 hours after MI and lasting
more than 15 minutes will extend their infarction. Patients with recurrent chest pain
have been reported to have an annual mortality in excess of 30%. Present evidence
does not support the use of thrombolytic agents for unstable angina but they are
indicated for recurrent infarction. Whether they should be used for recurrent
impending infarction within a few days of first infarction is unknown. Late thrombolysis is attended by increased risks of cardiac rupture and stroke and this must be
weighed against the theoretical benefits.

In patients who fail to respond to medical therapy, angiography and possible
PTCA or surgery should be performed. However, in patients who settle on medical
therapy, retrospective analysis has suggested that prognosis is no different with the
medical or surgical approach. It has been argued that the surgically treated patients
have less angina at outpatient follow-up; the patient on medical therapy, however,
always has the option of surgery at this time.

Exertional angina

Properly designed randomized studies show that there is no prognostic value in carrying out angiography and intervention routinely after MI, whether or not the exercise test is positive.

However, in patients with a positive exercise test at low level, or who have dis-
abling angina despite medical therapy, angiography should be carried out if the
patient is a candidate for intervention, as these patients have not been specifically
studied in the surgical trials; they have a worse prognosis and many will benefit
from coronary interventions by an improvement in symptoms. If the pattern of disease or the patient's symptoms warrant it, PTCA or surgery should be performed.
Although surgery in the first 48 hours after MI carries a relatively low risk, risk
increases in the following few weeks as the infarcted area of myocardium undergoes
liquefaction. The surgical dangers of damaging the friable myocardium may be considerable. For these reasons, surgery should be delayed where possible, and PTCA
may have a valuable role in helping to achieve this.

Arrhythmias

A beta blocker, amiodarone and electrical cardioversion are adequate to deal with
most problems.

Atrial fibrillation

The goals of therapy are to control rate, restore sinus rhythm (the spontaneous conversion rate is high) and prevent emboli. For patients with short bursts of atrial fibrillation a beta blocker will control rate and reduce episodes. For patients with sustained atrial fibrillation, beta blockers may control rate but amiodarone probably achieves a more rapid and higher rate conversion to sinus rhythm. A major disadvantage of amiodarone, if it needs to be given rapidly, is the requirement to give it via a central line. Digoxin has little role to play in the control of atrial fibrillation in this setting, being slow to gain control of rate and relatively ineffective in restoring sinus rhythm. If atrial fibrillation causes severe haemodynamic compromise, electrical cardioversion may be warranted.

Supraventricular tachycardia with bundle-branch block is over-diagnosed in the post-infarction patient. Treatment of ventricular tachycardia with intravenous verapamil can be disastrous. Adenosine can be used to help differentiate supraventricular from ventricular tachycardia. However, amiodarone is appropriate regardless of the origin of the arrhythmia.

Ventricular tachycardia or fibrillation

If haemodynamic collapse ensues then electrical cardioversion is required.

If ventricular tachycardia is sustained and the patient is not severely compromised, then amiodarone is probably the safest and most effective drug but needs to be given centrally. Class I agents used singly may also be effective but can cause haemodynamic compromise, especially if used in combination or rapid succession. Cardioversion is preferable to the administration of multiple agents. The role of magnesium, outside the setting of *torsades de pointes*, is unclear.

Frequent or complex ventricular extrasystoles are associated with a worse prognosis even after correcting for the fact that they often reflect poorer ventricular function. No specific anti-arrhythmic treatment is indicated at present but, in view of the poorer prognosis, there is a strong case for treating with a beta blocker and, if ventricular function is compromised, an ACE inhibitor.

Sinus bradycardia

Sinus bradycardia rarely requires treatment. Reduce or stop bradycardic therapies if the rate is below 50 per minute. Dobutamine may be used to reverse bradycardia associated with beta blockade.

Second- and third-degree heart block

Prognosis is relatively good whether or not the patient is paced if the infarct is inferior, and poor whether or not the patient is paced if the infarct is anterior. Anterior infarcts causing conduction problems are usually large. If the ventricular rate is above 50/minute and the blood pressure adequate, then no pacing is required with inferior infarcts. If the rate is slower atropine should be given initially. Anterior infarcts with

conduction defects have a poor prognosis and, although of no proven benefit, pacing
is commonly recommended if any significant conduction abnormality develops.

Heart failure

Cause of heart failure should be determined (usually by echocardiography) rather
than assumed. Even severe mitral regurgitation may be inaudible after MI [4,5].
Heart failure developing during an evolving infarct is probably best treated with
intravenous nitrates and, if pulmonary oedema is present or incipient, diuretics.
These patients should also receive an ACE inhibitor once the infarction appears completed. Patients developing heart failure later in the course of infarction should be
treated with an ACE inhibitor with or without diuretics as necessary.

Cardiogenic shock

Causes of cardiogenic shock are severe left ventricular dysfunction, ventricular septal
rupture, severe mitral regurgitation (may be inaudible), cardiac rupture, right ventricular infarction or iatrogenic (beta blockade, verapamil, class I anti-arrhythmic agent).

The diagnosis can be resolved by echocardiography, and pressure and saturations
(for ventricular septal defect) in the pulmonary artery. Pulmonary artery pressure
monitoring is required for active management. Intra-aortic balloon pump should not
be instituted unless an attempt at a corrective procedure is going to be tried.

Treatment of cardiogenic shock
• Withdraw offending drugs

• Specific antidote
    beta blockade — dobutamine
    verapamil — calcium chloride

• Right ventricular infarct   dobutamine/dopamine and fluid load

• Left ventricular dysfunction
    dobutamine/dopamine (though no real evidence that it makes a difference to outcome)
    consider whether PTCA or surgery possible (if so, consider intra-aortic balloon pump)

• Cardiac rupture   pericardiocentesis/immediate surgery

• VSD or mitral regurgitation
    renal dose dopamine
    nitrate/nitroprusside if pressure not too low; if surgical candidate, consider intra-aortic
      balloon pump

Table 4.7. PTCA, percutaneous transluminal coronary angioplasty; VSD, ventricular septal defect.

Treatment depends on the underlying cause (*see* Table 4.7). Surgery should not be deferred if decided upon.

One short report [6] suggested that ACE inhibitors may be beneficial in cardiogenic shock. This awaits confirmation.

Ventricular septal defect (VSD)/mitral regurgitation

• If major haemodynamic compromise, treat as for cardiogenic shock.

•If no major haemodynamic compromise, treat as for patients with ventricular dysfunction.

Pericarditis/Dressler's syndrome

Painless pericarditis requires no specific treatment. Indomethacin can cause salt and water retention and heart failure, and may have a deleterious interaction with ACE inhibitors on renal function. Moreover, animal experiments suggest that indomethacin may have adverse effects on infarct scar formation. In pericarditis associated with pain, cautious use of indomethacin is warranted. In patients with relatively painless pericarditis and fever, paracetamol may be used to reduce fever if necessary. There seems little benefit in treating the raised erythrocyte sedimentation rate or anaemia associated with Dressler's syndrome. Steroids are rarely required.

Ventricular thrombus

Identification of left ventricular thrombus increases the risk of embolic events, but the majority of thrombi resolve without sequelae. Surgery is rarely indicated but is sometimes necessary if the thrombus is very labile; most thrombi are sessile. Patients who have had left ventricular thrombus identified should be anticoagulated with heparin and then warfarin. There is a reasonable argument for life-long anticoagulation but it should certainly be continued for 6–8 weeks [1,7–10].

Summary

Although the large clinical trials have increased the scientific basis for the management of MI, they have also enhanced the art of medicine. The trials tell us only general truths. The art of medicine is required to adapt what is true, in general, to individual patients.

A major beneficial role for only five classes of agents has been established for use after MI: thrombolytics, antithrombotics (aspirin/warfarin), bradycardic agents (beta blockers/verapamil), lipid-lowering agents and ACE inhibitors. However, we may be at only the beginning of the ACE inhibitor era. If studies such as QUIET show that ACE inhibitors favourably modify the natural history of atheroma even in patients with good ventricular function, this will imply that all patients should be treated with an ACE inhibitor after an MI indefinitely.

References

1. Jugdutt BI *et al.* **Prospective two-dimensional echocardiographic evaluation of left ventricular thrombus and embolism after acute myocardial infarction.** *J Am Coll Cardiol* 1989, **13**:554–564.

2. Malmberg *et al.*: **Diabetes Insulin Glucose Acute Myocaridal Infarction (DIGAMI) Study.** *(J Am Coll Cardiol, in press 1995).*

3. Lapinleimu H *et al.*: **Prospective trial in 1062 infants of diet low in saturated fat and cholesterol.** *Lancet* 1995, **345**:471–476.

4. Tcheng JE *et al.*: **Outcome of patients sustaining acute ischaemic mitral regurgitation during myocardial infarction.** *Ann Intern Med* 1992, **117**:18–24.

5. Lehmann KG *et al.*: **Mitral regurgitation in early myocardial infarction. Incidence, clinical detection and prognostic implications.** *Ann Intern Med* 1992, **117**:10–17.

6. Lipkin DP *et al*: **Beneficial effect of captopril in cardiogenic shock** [letter]. *Lancet* 1987, **2**:327.

7. Halperin JL, Fuster V: **Left ventricular thrombus and stroke after myocardial infarction: toward prevention or perplexity?** *J Am Coll Cardiol* 1989, **14**:912–914.

8. Johannessen K-A *et al*: **Usefulness of aspirin plus dipyridamole in reducing left ventricular thrombus formation in anterior wall acute myocardial infarction.** *Am J Cardiol* 1989, **63**:101–102.

9. Kupper AJF *et al*: **Effect of low dose acetylsalicylic acid on the frequency and hematologic activity of left ventricular thrombus in anterior wall acute myocardial infarction.** *Am J Cardiol* 1989, **63**:917–918.

10. Vecchio C *et al* (GISSI-2 connected study): **Left ventricular thrombus in anterior acute myocardial infarction after thrombolysis.** *Circulation* 1991, **84**:512–519.

Index